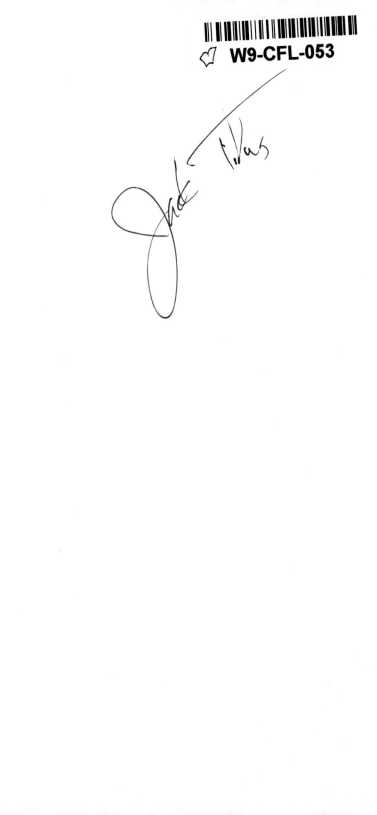

STRO_2KE

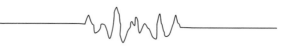

STRO_2KE:
Recovery with Oxygen

by Polly Houston

Best Publishing Company

Design by   Jill McAdoo
                 Rebecca Henestofel

Cover by   Rebecca Henestofel

Edited by   James T. Joiner
                 Joel F. Russell

ISBN No: 1-930536-21-6

Library of Congress catalog number: 2003112768

Best Publishing Company
2355 North Steves Boulevard
P.O. Box 30100
Flagstaff, Arizona 86003-0100 USA

To John
For his unswerving love,
patience, and belief in the project.

Two roads diverged in a wood, and I –
I took the one less traveled by,
And that has made all the difference.
                    —Robert Frost

Table of contents

x

1

IT'S ONLY A "MINOR" STROKE

On a gray November morning, my husband was already up. He's probably in the kitchen, I thought, glancing at the clock. Seven o'clock: time to get moving. I rolled out of bed and started toward the bathroom, but something was wrong. When I got to my feet, I was so unsteady that I had to clutch at a chair to keep from falling, and I grabbed the dresser as I passed it. This is ridiculous, I thought. I guess I'm not quite awake yet. But I was awake, and I remembered the odd, slightly disorganized feeling I'd had the day before. Well, that was yesterday. Today was a new day, and I was going to walk normally as I started back to the bedroom.

I didn't get very far.

My right leg gave way. Just folded under me.

I still don't understand why I wasn't frightened when I landed on the floor and lay in a twisted heap. I didn't struggle to get up. Didn't even wonder why I'd fallen.

Instead, I was flooded with an overwhelmingly peaceful sense of acceptance, an inner "knowing" that I shouldn't get up. Shouldn't even try, so I simply lay on the floor, placidly curled in a little ball and waited for John, my husband.

He was horrified when he saw me, repeating over and over, "Polly, what's wrong? What are you doing?"

1

"It's all right," I answered calmly, as if I usually lay in a heap on the floor. "There's nothing to worry about. I think maybe I'm just having a little stroke."

If I'd known then what a "little" stroke meant, I don't think I could have faced the future.

My doctor had recently scolded me because my cholesterol and blood pressure were a bit high, but the numbers were only moderately above normal, so I hadn't been frightened. I obediently took the pills he'd prescribed and occasionally exercised, but other than that I more or less ignored the problem. I knew absolutely nothing about strokes although I did know that high blood pressure is a cautionary signal.

John and I knew that people are told to go to the hospital when they have a stroke, but neither of us knew why. What could the hospital do? I had just had an unusual minor accident, but I wasn't ill. I felt no pain. I had no problem except the mysterious collapse of my right leg, and I was sure I would recover in a week or so. I always heal quickly. I didn't know that strokes are progressive, that they don't just "happen all at once" like a broken bone. Neither of us knew that there is a three-hour time constraint for treatment, and we had no idea that the original problem, a very small blood clot that had blocked an artery in my brain, was just the beginning of a series of crippling events.

John helped me to my feet and steadied me as I limped back to sit on the bed. He brought me a glass of orange juice and in a voice filled with concern asked, "Should I call 9-1-1? Ask for an ambulance?" I scoffed at the thought of an ambulance. Why pay the $750 charge that had recently been discussed in our local newspaper? I should have known that senior citizens who take a tumble are advised to always request an ambulance. A fall can break a fragile bone, and improper lifting or heaving can do additional damage to the fallen senior or to the person doing the lifting. I knew I hadn't broken a bone. I had no bumps or bruises. I'd fallen in slow motion. "No way," I insisted, wanting to be sensible and kind to the family budget. "Not for a short, three-mile ride to the hospital."

Wrong.

I was so very wrong.

We should have acted immediately.

Since that morning, I've learned that Medicare helps seniors pay their medical bills. The Medicare program covers much of the cost of an ambulance, and your health insurance probably covers the rest. But we didn't know. Nor did we know that the paramedics who staff an ambulance have been trained to recognize early stroke symptoms. And they know that possible stroke patients should be brought to a community Stroke Center, if one is available, or to a well-equipped regional hospital.

Instead of acting as if this were a medical emergency, I calmly sipped my juice while we waited until the doctor's office opened at 9:00 so we could ask the receptionist for advice. She didn't sound as if we were facing a medical emergency. She just told John to drive me to our local community hospital.

At our house, we take two daily newspapers, a weekly news magazine, and routinely watch the nightly news. In fact, we've been accused of being "news junkies." John is a retired professor of political science, and I'm a traditional wife and mother. We always thought we were reasonably well-informed about the world. Of course, we knew heart attacks must be treated immediately—we had read many articles describing cardiac problems and the ingenious new ways heart disease can be treated today. A number of our friends and relatives experienced heart problems and recovered. We've mourned the loss of a few who are no longer with us. Cancer was frequently in the medical news. I was very aware of breast cancer and the importance of a yearly mammogram.

But we'd read almost nothing about strokes. Nothing about warning symptoms; nothing that explained "why" they should be treated as quickly as possible. We didn't know strokes are so common that they are the third highest cause of death and the leading cause of crippling disabilities in the United States. I had heard whispered horror tales of people who had been felled by one, but those stories didn't apply to me. I was a healthy older woman, and I was feeling almost normal. This couldn't be serious.

We knew nothing, that is, other than one short paragraph in one of the recent newspapers announcing a new "miracle" drug for stroke treatment. Either the reporter had forgotten to mention or we failed to remember one small detail. The "miracle drug" can only be administered within the first three hours.

In addition to calling an ambulance immediately, what else should we have done that morning? At the very least, I should have taken a couple of aspirins the moment I even suspected that I might be having a stroke. Aspirin dissolves blood clots. In Great Britain, administering an aspirin is the immediate standard treatment of choice. Aspirin was recommended in the medical text I read many months later, and American physicians now agree that either aspirin or the blood-thinner Coumadin are useful, effective drugs for dissolving blood clots.

Although I've combed the Internet for stroke information, I've never seen vitamins recommended by any of the traditional doctors, but today I routinely take a daily B-complex capsule containing folic acid and B-12 to counteract possibly high homocysteine levels in my blood. And today, at the first hint that I might be having another stroke, I would take a couple of aspirins and gulp a bunch of antioxidants—C's, E's, etc., to counteract some that avalanche of enzymes and chemicals that I have now learned were beginning to flood my brain (see Chapters 6 and 7). Maybe antioxidants don't help, but then again, maybe they would be useful. This is not medical advice; I'm just telling you what I, as a lay person who has learned a lot about strokes, would do today.

But we didn't have a clue that morning.

I was still speaking as easily and coherently as I had for all of my seventy-seven years. I didn't have a headache. No nausea. No double vision. No pain. Just that unexpected weakness in my right leg and an ephemeral, unsteady, "spacey" sensation.

When friends have asked me, "What did it feel like when you had your stroke?" I've had to answer, "I honestly don't know."

I now believe I might have noticed the earliest symptoms the previous day, because I'd felt as if an unnamed, undefined "something" was wrong, but I'd ignored it. We all have days like that, although I remember thinking on my way to an appointment, "I must drive very carefully today because I feel odd, not quite right." My balance was just fine, but in the grocery store that day my right foot occasionally scuffed across the floor. I could "make" it walk normally, however, if I simply remembered to lift it.

Hindsight is so clear.

My body was trying to tell me something was wrong. But I didn't listen.

Didn't get the message.

That night when I went to sleep I thought, "I'll be okay in the morning."

Not so.

Because my first symptoms were so minor and so gradual, I suspect that I might have had a "traveling" clot—a cluster of cells that had clumped together and were squeezing through increasingly smaller capillaries in my brain until they clogged a tiny blood vessel. But even if I'd known then what I know now, I probably would have thought I was just having the usual vague "senior citizen" aches and pains.

Diagnosing a stroke isn't always easy, even for the professionals. Let me share a message I found months later on the Internet.

A stroke nurse was answering a stroke-survivor's questions.

The worst part about the three hour window is that both the patient and the staff need to be alert to the possibility that the patient actually IS having a stroke, because it takes up to three hours to run all the necessary tests to determine whether a clot or a bleed is causing the symptoms.

In the case of a bleed, it could be disastrous to give tPA (tissue Plasminogen Activator). But for a CLOT it can mean the difference between SEVERE FUNCTIONAL LOSSES and NO DISABILITY.

If an artery is bleeding, an angiogram can be used to identify the location and to outline steps to minimize the damage.

It all goes back to teaching the general public and giving the medical professionals sufficient time to conduct tests and administer drugs.

Not all stroke patients are over fifty and NOT ALL HAVE SUDDEN ONSETS. In fact, with a traveling clot, a gradual, step-wise progression is the norm.

It was almost 9:30 that morning when John helped me into my pink quilted housecoat and shabby, well-loved slippers and steadied me as we walked to the car. We drove to the hospital's Emergency entrance where he went in to ask for a wheelchair. The medical people were in no hurry either. Years later, I learned that the emergency room physician had actually been following one of the American Heart Association's recommended protocols for stroke treatment. After a leisurely CAT scan, an EKG, and a couple of blood tests, the on-duty doctor, with a casual, "Let's just watch and wait" attitude, decided my guess had been correct. "You haven't had a heart attack," he agreed. "What you've had is a minor stroke."

Remembering the recent story in our local newspaper, at that point I asked for the new wonder drug tPA that had been enthusiastically hailed as the new treatment, a "miraculous cure for strokes."

The physician shook his head. His response was curt. "Oh, no. We can't give you tPA. You don't know exactly what time you had your stroke, and it can only be given within three hours of the blockage. If we were to give it to you now, it could cause uncontrolled bleeding. Maybe even kill you."

I later learned that administering the miraculous new clot-dissolving enzyme involves a complicated series of injections. Physicians are cautioned that it must only be administered within the first three hours of clot formation. Not only was I unable to give the doctor a precise time the stroke occurred, but the routine tests I was given in the hospital took longer than three hours. I sensed that the emergency doctor wasn't enthusiastic about the drug. Later, I wondered if he even knew very much about strokes.

I was given absolutely no medication, not even an aspirin. I couldn't help wondering, "what's the point of coming to the hospital? Very expensive if all you get is food and a bed." I now realize, of course, that I was under medical observation while my stroke was "developing," and I was available several days later when another physician decided to run some additional tests.

I've been told recently that when tPA was first announced with great fanfare in the press, our local physicians met to discuss the new drug. They agreed it was expensive (rumor says a thousand dollars), that it doesn't always work, and it could be dangerous. The doctors in our area decided they would not use tPA. However, as of today, tissue plasminogen activator is still the only drug recommended for stroke treatment by the Stroke Council, a division of the American

Heart Association. As you'll see throughout this book, many newer, more effective treatments and drugs have been approved by the US Food and Drug Administration, and I've read reports noting tPA is not always effective, even when administered within the three-hour time frame.

I'd felt so safe, so secure when I'd asked for science's latest miracle cure, but when the emergency physician refused to administer the new drug, I didn't know enough to be frightened. I felt drowsy, but serene, with a child-like sense of acceptance— probably the result of that wave of biochemicals that were flooding my brain. I've heard my state of mind described as "la-la land." It was a very pleasant feeling, and I was still sure I'd be home within a couple of days.

"Don't worry," the doctor said with a paternalistic pat on my shoulder, "It's only a minor stroke," as he dismissed me and sent me to a bed in the patients' area of the hospital.

STROKE: RECOVERY WITH OXYGEN

2

MY HOSPITAL EXPERIENCE

"Well," I thought after I'd been safely tucked into a hospital bed, "That wasn't too bad. Now, let's get on with taking care of the problem. That's what I'm here for, isn't it?"

"What happens next?"

I had my first clue that all was NOT fine when I said to the nice male nurse who'd helped me get settled, "I skipped breakfast this morning. Is it too late for lunch or a snack of some sort?" I wasn't really hungry, but it was now the middle of the afternoon and I thought I ought to behave as if this was just a normal day. He looked a bit startled, and said, "Sure. No problem." He quickly returned with a full meal. Then, he proceeded to cut up the meat on my plate as if he were preparing it for a very small child.

Now it was my turn to be startled. I'd cut their food into bite-sized pieces when my children were toddlers, but that was many years ago. Did this friendly man think I wasn't capable of eating like a normal adult? Oh, well. The last time I'd been in a hospital for any reason other than visiting a sick friend was decades ago. Maybe hospitals are different today. I thanked him and politely reached for my fork as if I were accustomed to having someone cut up my food.

Oops. Something wasn't working.

All my life, I've been right handed. My right arm made all the right moves, but I couldn't open my hand. What was this? My fingers were working normally this morning when I drank a glass of orange juice. Now, I couldn't pick up the fork; my hand wouldn't open. Aware of sympathy in the nurse's eyes, I managed to stuff the fork into my fist and stab at the food. For some reason, the fork didn't always find my mouth. Eating my first post-stroke meal was not a pretty sight.

And there were more surprises.

Like that little matter of the bathroom. As instructed, I punched the red button attached to my bed to ask for help when I felt nature's call. My, how hospitals have changed. Nowadays they use a two-way communication system. The patient pushes a button, and a disembodied voice in the wall asks, "What do you want?" You're supposed to tell the wall what you need. Sooner or later a nurse will arrive.

Ten minutes later a nurse walked in carrying a bedpan. "Next time," she said cheerfully, "let's try to walk to the bathroom. You don't want to turn into a couch potato." When she retrieved the bedpan, I was shocked by the smell. Yuck! My urine smelled vile. Stinky urine. That was odd. Months later, I learned that a cascade of destructive fluids and enzymes had been flooding my brain, killing many brain cells during the active phase of the stroke. I think my kidneys were valiantly working overtime, attempting to filter the sludge of dead cells and corrosive biochemicals from my blood.

Later, after I'd learned there were at least two kinds of strokes, I asked my doctor what kind of stroke

12

I'd had. He told me it was a small clot, or an infarct. Briefly, that means that a cluster of cells stick together in a clump, forming a clot in the blood; the clot floats along in the blood stream until it dissolves, unless it gets stuck in one of the capillaries that feed the brain. When one of the brain's tiny capillaries becomes blocked, it swells, and the swelling squeezes any nearby blood vessels. It is that secondary squeezing by a blocked capillary that creates most of a stroke's damage.

The human brain, the creator of our every thought, every skill and memory, the center of our very "self," is also the mastermind controlling every organ, every nerve, muscle, and bone in the body. This amazing super-computer only weighs about three pounds. There is no extra space inside our tightly packed skulls, so when a single capillary is squeezed, that blood vessel swells, restricting the delivery of oxygen to the cells it feeds. Without a normal supply of blood, those brain cells go to sleep, or as one researcher says, they "become dormant." (For a complete description of this process, see Chapter 7.)

I had no hint of the disaster that was, at that moment, going on inside my head. I was not frightened. I just felt drowsy and so tranquil.

For the rest of that first afternoon, I massaged my closed-up fist and managed to uncurl my right hand, one finger at a time until I could wiggle each finger on command as if I were typing or playing scales on a piano. By bedtime my hand was working almost normally.

But I hadn't tried to walk. I believed my body was working reasonably well. I watched a little TV after a light supper and thought, "What's the big deal about strokes?" before I dropped off to sleep.

The next morning was something else. When I tried to get out of bed, I was shocked to find that I'd lost my sense of balance. I couldn't stand without help. And my right leg didn't work. I could not force my leg to move when a nurse came to help me.

And that morning I couldn't open my hand again. I'd thought I'd fixed the problem the day before, but I absolutely could not make those fingers move. I massaged my hand all morning just as I'd successfully done yesterday, but nothing happened today. Not a flicker.

Strangely enough, I was still serenely accepting everything that was happening with a child-like sense of, "It's okay. This will all go away in a day or so." I didn't have the slightest clue to the fact that a stroke doesn't happen all at once, that the damage is progressive. Today, I believe I was being calmed by nature's tranquilizer—that flood of destructive, caustic biochemicals that were still at work, killing additional brain cells.

On the second or third day in the hospital, one of the physicians from my regular doctor's office walked into my room and greeted me with a cheerful, "You are so lucky, Polly. We'll have you back on skis in a couple of weeks."

"Sounds great," I quipped. "I've never learned to ski."

I still don't know why he said I was lucky, unless he couldn't face the devastating aftermath of a stroke for

14

someone he knew. Or, unless the clot had just missed a vital area in my brain—one that would have killed me. I do know he was trying to cheer me up and it worked. I was comforted.

The hospital kept me for a week. Over the next few days, laboratory technicians took many additional blood samples, and a machine tested me for arterial blockages. When I asked, the technician said the left artery running from my heart up through my neck was 70 percent blocked. Nobody seemed to think that was unusual or dangerous.

I was still speaking easily. John spent the days in my room, entertaining me by reading aloud, or we idly conversed. That was nice for me, and no problem for the staff—one of the joys of a small, community hospital.

I was given no medications. No neuroprotectants. No oxygen. Not so much as an aspirin. With persistent massage, my right hand did limber up a bit during the day, but my balance did not improve, not even with a nurse firmly holding my shoulder.

When I met my first physical therapist, I stared in disbelief at the narrow little belt she tied around my waist. I was sure her two-inch-wide strip of fabric would be useless, but it did keep me from toppling over. With her at my side and that belt around my waist for balance, I was able to walk—sort of. I managed to make my right leg move and was able to wobble as far as the end of the hall and back again.

My next helper was also a physical therapist, although she was active in a different "specialty." I learned there is a strict division in the therapy world between those who work on legs and walking, and those who work on arms and upper body movements. I had a nice conversation with an occupational therapist (they teach stroke patients to eat, with emphasis on safe swallowing) and a speech therapist. Some were more more pleasant than others.

"Come on. You can do it. Lift that thumb," the cute little blonde with a nerve-grating, false-cheerful chirp ordered several days later. Obediently, I gritted my teeth, took a deep breath, and tried again, hoping to placate her. I knew she was trying to help me. Nothing. Yesterday I'd been able to force my right thumb to lift a half inch, just one time, before the muscles refused to obey. Not this day. "Try again," she commanded. So I took another deep breath and set my jaw. This time I would move that thumb. Not a quiver. With every ounce of strength I possessed, my brain shouted, "Move!" The muscles in my forearm shook. Mentally I heaved and strained. Still nothing. The electrical circuits in my brain just weren't working.

Could they be gone for good?

Now I was getting worried. Maybe a stroke, even a "minor" stroke, really was a big deal.

After I'd been declared "out of danger" (read that as "stroke completed"), I was sent to a nursing/convalescent facility where I spent two weeks. With hours of physical therapy each day, I graduated from a wheelchair to a walker, to depending on a cane for balance, but my muscles were so weak.

My balance was weird. I felt "tippy," as if my body had forgotten the difference between backward and forward.

I was discovering new problems with my right arm as well. Brushing my teeth was now almost impossible. I could open my right hand once again, but I could not force that right arm to move back and forth in the old, familiar rhythm. I was reduced to "brushing" my teeth by moving my head left and right across the toothbrush; my mouth was beginning to feel like a fur-lined cave.

Maybe in the stroke world, mine was really was considered "minor." I had no trouble swallowing, my eyes were working very well, and my digestive system didn't know anything was wrong. When a speech therapist gave me a simple test requiring picture comprehension, we decided "that" part of my brain was still okay, but I honestly didn't know enough to celebrate. I had not yet learned about speech confusion or language problems.

The old phrase, "Different strokes for different folks," now holds a world of new meaning for me. Some stroke victims are forced to exist on baby food because they've lost control of their "swallow" muscles. Others are left with speech problems (aphasia— "doctor-speak" for not being able to find the word you want). I know one stroke survivor who is unable to pronounce the word he is trying to say, but he can spell it. That's an example of the brain's compartmentalization. I had no double vision. I could still see perfectly well to read, but I was too weak to hold a book. Why was I weak? All I'd been doing for three weeks was just lying in bed.

"How long is this going to last?" I finally asked my primary-care physician.

He didn't look at me. Didn't exactly answer my question. "We don't know why you had a stroke," he said, staring intently at my chart. "It's just one of those things." I've since learned that his evasive answer is absolutely standard.

He tried to look as neutral as possible when I pressed him. "But when am I going to get better?"

He didn't actually say, "Never. Part of your brain has been hopelessly destroyed," but now I know that is what he'd been taught in medical school. That is what he believed.

But his information was not totally correct. So much has been learned about the brain in the last 20–30 years.

After I was discharged from the convalescent hospital and was home again, physical therapists visited me twice a week for a month. I was given another two months of outpatient therapy in our valley's large regional hospital. I certainly wasn't functioning like my old self, but I was now able to walk, so the physical therapist told me I was no longer a danger to myself or others in the community. That's the cut-off point.

Slowly and reluctantly, I began to understand that I now was a handicapped person and would be for the rest of my life.

Six months later I was driving again, because my reflexes were still intact, my vision was normal, and I could trust my good left hand, arm, and foot. Driving is essential in our small town. The nearest public transportation is a mile and a half from our house, down a very steep hill. In case you're wondering, I recently passed a "Medical Reevaluation" exam given by the Oregon Department of Transportation and my driver's license was renewed. The exam was complete with questions about my medications, vision, mental competence, the rules of the road, and a driving test.

I now treasure my blue "handicapped" parking card because I, who used to love the mountains and hiking Oregon's trails, became exhausted after limping three short blocks.

Slowly, my brain began to rewire itself. My right hand was still very clumsy, but my teeth were shiny-clean after I switched to an electric toothbrush. My husband and I were still able to live independently. I could manage the washing machine and dryer, shop for groceries and do basic cooking, and we hired a lady to vacuum the house and clean the kitchen and bathroom every two weeks. What more did I want? I desperately wanted to get back to being a normal non-handicapped person.

One of the minor hassles of post-stroke life has been losing my ability to write. I'd never realized what a vital role casual scribbling plays in our lives. It was humiliating to have to say, "Oh, I can't write," when I was asked to jot down a telephone number, fill out a simple form at the dentist's office, to rent a videotape, or dash off a short note.

I was horrified the first time I tried to write my name. The therapist laid a 9 x 12 sheet of paper on the dining room table, handed me a pencil and told me to write "P-o-l-l-y." It was hard to believe what my hand produced. Those five letters filled the entire sheet of paper and they looked like jagged streaks of lightning. I guess my brain was trying to cobble together the missing electrical connections, but my fingers didn't get the message. The "writing" I produced when I laboriously pressed the pencil to the paper could be compared to routing a telephone call to a friend next door, but the damaged telephone system (my brain) had apparently tried to connect the call by sending it from Ashland to New Orleans, then to Hong Kong and back across the Atlantic Ocean to France, across the Pacific once again to Japan, and on to New York before it finally succeeded in linking me up with my next-door neighbor.

I stared at the mess, trying not to weep. Do you have any idea how many times a day someone asks you to "just jot something down"? To "sign this"? Every time you use a credit card and a zillion other places. I was able to type (left handed) checks for birthday presents to the grandchildren and for grocery money, and I could laboriously draw something that the bank teller was willing to accept as my new signature, but she knew me. And she knew I'd had a stroke.

Jane, my oldest daughter, is a medical researcher, so I'd asked her to search the Internet for "stroke" information because I wanted to understand why I was still having these problems. It was hard for me to believe, but it was true when she said she'd found almost nothing except the usual warnings: Don't smoke. Keep your weight down and your blood pressure low. Stay as active as possible. If you do become a stroke victim, beware of depression.

Ha! Those words were not "funny ha ha." They were downright discouraging.

Who wouldn't be depressed when twenty-four hours of every day, everything you do, every movement you try to make is either very laborious or totally blocked, and you've finally realized you are never going to recover?

20

3

Life after a "minor" stroke

Two years later I was turning into a frustrated, angry, depressed woman. I'd been faithfully doing the exercises the therapists had recommended, but I was still handicapped. Yes, I could limp a few wobbly blocks without a cane. The darned thing had tripped me a time or two so I gave it away, but I wasn't really "walking." I could not make my legs move properly. My left leg moved the way it had always moved, but try as hard as I could, my right leg would not cooperate—it was still stiff and slow. My body had lost its natural rhythm and my balance was still unsteady—that backward-and-forward tippy feeling had not gone away.

I continued to ask myself, why? How I hated being handicapped! My right hand was still almost useless, I was tired all the time and felt horrible, as if my nerves were grating against each other like fingernails scraped across a blackboard.

"Exercise," the therapists had stressed, so I was swimming every day. At first I'd been exhilarated to find that I could actually walk with a slow, but even, stride while I was in the pool. The water steadied me as I cruised back and forth across the shallow end. The therapy was helping me regain a bit of control, because many months later I was actually swimming, although all I could manage was a stately, lop-sided breast-stroke.

My right side was still so badly out of sync with my left that all I got was a faceful of water every time I tried a normal stroke. My arms, like my legs, absolutely refused to move in the old, familiar rhythm.

I was driving again. My sight and reflexes were intact and I could depend on my sturdy left side. I was able to prepare our simple meals and could manage the washing machine and dryer. We were still living in our own home, taking care of ourselves. What more did I want?

I wanted to feel alive again. Not constantly struggling on the ragged edge.

To feel like a whole person.

And I wanted an explanation. Why wasn't I regaining my lost abilities? I now realized that a stroke, even a minor one, was a *VERY* big deal. I wholeheartedly agreed with the expert who'd written, "an untreated stroke always leaves the victim with varying degrees of disability." If I wasn't ever going to recover, there was nothing I could do but accept it. Just doggedly go on breathing. But if there was any way I could regain my "real" life, I wanted to know about it. I was determined to find out the answer and do it.

So I went looking.

Why was it so hard to find any information about strokes? The first thing I learned was that cardiovascular disease is called a "cardiovascular accident" (CVA), and it kills one out of every two men and women in our "advanced" industrial nation. Every authority agreed on one dismal fact—strokes are the leading cause for crippling disabilities. So why wasn't anyone talking about strokes or writing about them?

I'd seen plenty of public service ads discussing heart ailments on television and the radio. Our local bookstores and the public library offered hundreds of heart-healthy cookbooks and advice about heart disease—how to recognize a heart attack, how to avoid one, how to recover from one. There were always heart-related diet and exercise stories in the popular magazines. Our newspapers were full of articles describing the latest miracle drug, or operation, or some new device to help a failing heart. And, of course, on television there was more information than I ever wanted to know about acid reflux disease (heartburn) and infected toenails, but not a word about strokes.

Despite a still-clumsy right hand, after six months I had improved enough to be able to use my trusty old Macintosh. I began searching the Internet, determined to learn everything I could about this disaster that had changed my life.

I found this cheerful bit:

> *Stroke is the third leading cause of death, ranking just behind diseases of the heart and all forms of cancer. Strokes kill about 150,000 Americans every year and are the leading cause of serious, long-term disability. Roughly 750,000 people have a stroke each year. About 500,000 are first-ever strokes.*
>
> *Approximately 4,400,000 stroke victims are alive today.*
>
> *One third of those who suffer a stroke don't survive the initial attack. Another third have to enter nursing homes. Only one-third improve, and many of these patients are left with disabilities that hinder their ability to resume their pre-stroke lives.*
>
> Alternative Medicine, Issue 15

I stared at the numbers.

Seven hundred and fifty thousand strokes a year! Strokes are *THAT* common!

If strokes kill a hundred thousand people a year and damage hundreds of thousands more, why aren't they ever mentioned in the news? Of course I knew heart attacks are the number one cause of death. The Heart Association has done a great job of alerting Americans to the perils of cholesterol-clogged arteries and a sedentary lifestyle, of the benefits of a low-salt, low-fat diet. I've walked on Heart Walks for years and sent checks to help fund heart research.

And of course I knew the dreaded "Big C" is our number two killer. I've gone on many a walk for breast cancer awareness and for cancer research.

But strokes are our nation's number three killer!

Before I became one of those unhappy four and a half million men, women, and children living with stroke damage, I'd had no idea they were so common. I am not alone. Just last week I met a woman who asked what I was working on. "A book about strokes, because I had one." My answer surprised her. "Really? When I was a girl I knew lots of people who'd had a stroke, but today I never hear of one. I thought there was some new treatment that meant they'd almost been eliminated."

"You're right, but you're also wrong," I agreed. "It's sad, but very true. We seldom hear strokes mentioned today, and I don't understand, because they have *NOT* been almost eliminated. In fact, medical experts are saying the number of strokes is *increasing* every year. I've read that today, in the U.S., someone will have a stroke every fifty-three seconds.

That means more than a stroke a minute, every day, 365 days a year. Even those numbers are going to climb (the experts tell us) as the baby-boomers enter their fifties."

We both shook our heads, puzzled by the silent treatment.

After I'd asked my daughter to send me any stroke information she could find, I'd been a bit skeptical when she said she'd seen almost nothing. Now that I was looking for myself, I realized she was right. There were no books about strokes. Amazon.com didn't list a single "stroke" title. I could find nothing about strokes in the popular magazines. There was not a word in the newspapers, not even any upbeat stories about stroke research. Apparently no one, except the hundreds of thousands of people living stroke-damaged lives, was interested in this all-too-common problem.

And why should they be?

Everyone knows you are born with every brain cell you will ever have. *Everyone knows* stroke victims just become vegetables, and nothing can be done except "keep them alive" and try to help and comfort their hard-pressed caregivers.

Sometimes, what everyone knows is just plain wrong.

I found one researcher who had written:

> *Most otherwise healthy stroke victims will live another ten or twenty years, struggling every day to achieve as normal a life as possible.*

This was a truly devastating bit of news if it meant that the odd, vaguely disorganized feeling I'd noticed so many months ago, and a right foot that had dragged slightly while I was shopping in a grocery store, had condemned me to another ten or twenty years of this exhausting, frustrating life.

This isn't living. This is just existing.

Maybe it was because the Internet itself was still relatively new, but every time I asked my computer to look up "stroke," "brain attack," or "CVA" (cerebral vascular accident)—every stroke word or phrase I could think of to explain *why* I wasn't recovering—the American Heart Association's stroke page popped up, along with the same useless, bland, generalized information Jane had already sent to me. There were warnings about depression and words of encouragement for the caregivers. There was nothing that explained why I was still crippled.

I couldn't find any information about that unsteady, backward-and-forward, almost out-of-control balance problem I was constantly fighting. No reason or explanation was given for those rigid, spastic muscles that were making my daily life—simple things like getting dressed, eating, even speaking—so difficult. No explanation for my ever-present fatigue or the constant frustration of a clumsy body that now resisted making ordinary movements, things the body had always done so effortlessly. Nothing to explain the damaged "wiring" in my body.

No wonder I was frustrated. Angry. This information "black hole" almost guaranteed *depression*.

Then former President Gerald Ford had a stroke.

Until his well-publicized stroke, the media had apparently decided that strokes weren't worth mentioning. But Gerald Ford had been the President of the United States, so his stroke was "news."

Tom Brokaw's statistics are meticulously checked by staff members so when he told us that seven hundred and fifty thousand Americans would be felled by a stroke this year—someone every fifty-three seconds—I agreed with him. Yes, I thought, seven hundred fifty thousand is a very hefty number indeed.

The reporter said President Ford had been noticing vague symptoms when he checked into a hospital, and had been sent home. The doctors told him he probably was just overtired or maybe he had a touch of the "flu." He was back the next day with slurred speech and stroke symptoms that were far more severe than mine. Surely he'd gone past that short three-hour "window of opportunity" allowed by tPA—the American Heart Association's favorite remedy. How could President Ford have walked out of the hospital "completely recovered" several days later while I, just an ordinary American housewife with far less severe symptoms, who'd checked into the hospital much more quickly, was now a permanently disabled person?

What was the difference? I knew President Ford was older than me. He'd played a lot of golf, but so had I. Was he healthier? Or had he been treated more effectively? Had his physicians used surgery or off-label drugs that our local doctors were either not aware of or just failed to use? You will find in later chapters that I've learned the brain needs oxygen. Without it, brain cells die, and I've learned there are surgeries and stents that can deliver a supply of oxygen-rich blood to the brain. I'm happy for Gerald Ford that he had a "complete recovery." But I'm envious. The after-effects of an untreated stroke are extremely unpleasant.

Our former president's experience did point up two important facts for those of us who are neither prominent nor well-informed:

(1) At the first hint that you might be having a stroke you should request an ambulance because the paramedics will take a suspected stroke patient to a "Primary Stroke Center" instead of delivering the patient to a general-purpose community hospital. Strokes can be very hard to diagnose, so don't wait for things to get worse. Even former President Ford's stroke was not identified at first.

(2) Because strokes are the third most common cause of death and the leading cause of permanent disability, it is important that the medical community take them seriously. According to the American Stroke Association, a "Primary Stroke Center" should be an essential part of every regional hospital, staffed by personnel who have been trained in stroke management. Twenty-four hour, seven day laboratory testing must be available.

Here's what I did find in 1997:

> *We must deliver the message that stroke is a medical emergency that needs to be viewed and treated with the same urgency as a heart attack.*
> The Brain Attack Coalition, 1995

But today strokes still spell "defeat" for many in the medical community. No wonder my primary-care physician was so evasive. The author of an editorial printed in the Journal of the American Medical Association (JAMA) writes:

> *Older practitioners will recall the days when patients with stroke were either treated at home or admitted to the hospital for compassionate observation. Neurologists made efforts to localize lesions and confirm functional areas of the brain and brainstem... Because the individual patient gained little, if anything, from these exercises, there was a public and professional aura of therapeutic helplessness surrounding stroke.*
>
> JAMA, vol. 283, No 23, June 21, 2000

Now I could understand the emergency room physician's "Let's just wait and see what happens" attitude.

The American Heart Association's Internet stroke page reported that a hemorrhagic stroke destroys such a large area of brain tissue that "nothing" can be done for hemorrhagic stroke victims. As you will read later in the book, the family members of some hemorrhagic stroke victims don't agree with this dark assessment.

I did find a short paragraph about transient ischemic attack (TIA)—temporary moments of confusion or dizziness that quickly disappear. The American Stroke Association authorities noted, "A TIA can be a warning of a possible stroke in the future," but nothing was said about what to do if you have a TIA other than the usual—get plenty of exercise, no smoking, and keep your weight and blood pressure down.

I did learn that 70 percent of strokes are ischemic (clot), and that there are two phases of an ischemic stroke—the acute phase which can last for eight or ten days, and the chronic stage, after a stroke has stabilized. The treatment for an "acute" stroke is different from that for a "chronic" patient.

I Meet Other Stroke Survivors

Strokes are not limited to sedentary senior citizens.

When I joined a "stroke chat-room," I learned that nobody is safe. A nurse wrote that she'd "stroked" at age forty-one. Another woman, a former aerobics instructor and body-builder who called herself a "health nut," told the group she'd been felled by a stroke on her forty-fifth birthday, and she said one of the women she'd met in the rehab hospital was under thirty. These stroke survivors hadn't been couch potatoes. They'd been leading physically active lives, weren't overweight, and had normal blood pressure.

People in their twenties and thirties have strokes, although the disaster is much more common in the forties crowd. Just yesterday I read this plaintive note in the chat-room:

Isn't there anyone young out there? I'm only 23.
You folks all seem to be so old—in your 40s and 50s.
I want to talk with someone my own age.

I was surprised and saddened to learn that children, even babies, can have strokes. One infant actually "stroked" before birth, and a five-year-old boy had suffered a massive stroke—half of his brain had been destroyed. I'm happy to add that his mother told the group that his young brain was rebuilding, and he is recovering nicely. This child's recovery is an encouraging example of the possibilities that stem-cell research may hold for all stroke victims in the future.

These people were tragic examples of lives unexpectedly damaged during their most productive years. Here are the thoughts of one 52-year-old man:

> *When I left the hospital it was very clear that the stroke had taken away my physical abilities as well as my identity as a provider, a professional consultant, and outdoor fanatic.*

This plucky guy was crediting much of his partial recovery to a martial arts therapy program he'd entered—a program designed by two black belt karate instructors after they had suffered strokes. Clearly, exercise doesn't prevent a stroke, but it does help in rehabilitation.

I thought about it, but didn't feel up to attempting karate at my age.

Many of the usual stroke-age grandmas and grandpas are now trapped in wheelchairs, condemned to be care receivers instead of caregivers, and it breaks their hearts.

How Much Had I Recovered after Six Months?

I could walk—a stiff right-leg-limp thanks to a set of spastic muscles, but without a cane. At mealtimes, the fork sometimes still twirled uselessly in my hand, and in spite of trying to be careful, I spilled food as awkwardly as a two-year-old. I could think clearly although my speech was slow, because of a few newly-rigid facial muscles. I had regained partial flexibility in my right hand, but brushing my teeth was still difficult. I couldn't use my right hand to write, not even my own name, but I could slowly type because I could make all but the two middle fingers of my right hand move more or less on command and they could find their proper place on a keyboard. Swimming was my daily exercise. The muscles on the right side of my face were flexible in the morning, but stiffened during the day. This made speaking, especially on the telephone, very difficult. Fortunately for me, my husband and my friends insisted that I try to live as normal a life as possible, and they ignored my limitations.

Common Stroke After-Effects

It could have been worse.

Some stroke survivors know what they want to say, but the wiring has been disconnected in their word-retrieval system (aphasia). They fumble for, but can't think of, a simple word like "window," a word they've been using all their lives. One fellow I've heard of is frequently unable to "say" a word, but he can spell it. I know a former librarian who has no trouble speaking, but he's been unable to read since his stroke. The letters, as symbols, don't make sense to him. This very bright man is now limited to watching the daily TV "soaps" to wile away the hours. That, I thought, is true frustration. How could he, or any of us who have been stroke-damaged, not be "depressed"?

Computers have opened new doors for many who had been living in a stroke-isolated world. People who had been stuck in lonely wheelchairs for many years can now "meet" other stroke victims and socialize, "talk" with their new friends. They share their lives, their joys and sorrows, and the names of medications they've found helpful. Some write of pain and name the painkillers that have helped. Others say their pain is unrelenting.

When I read their messages, I can almost believe that I really was lucky.

BUT I DON'T BELIEVE IT.

Isn't There Anything I Can Do to Recover?

I found something on the Internet about acupuncture being useful for stroke rehabilitation. There are three acupuncturists in town, so I called one and asked about his experience with stroke victims. "I've treated several," he said, "and it seemed to help them. Of course, I can't guarantee the results. All strokes are different."

Right. All strokes are different, but my primary care physician had agreed with the emergency room doctor that mine was only a "minor" stroke. It seemed worthwhile to give it a try.

My "minor" stroke must have been a lot more "major" than the doctors admitted, because after two months of weekly acupuncture treatments I felt only minor improvements. After all, the brain works by firing electrical impulses, and with more than ten billion neurons trying to send electrical messages on a scaffold of at least ten times ten billion glial cells, there must have been so many glitches in the wiring that acupuncture couldn't begin to reorganize everything for me.

True, there was that little matter of "pain" that the acupuncture eliminated. My right shoulder had been sore ever since the stroke. Not agonizing. It just ached, as if I'd slept on it wrong, and I couldn't raise my right arm higher than my shoulder. My doctor didn't seem concerned when I complained, but the acupuncturist listened very carefully, placed the needles in new places on my body—and I could raise that arm. The pain was gone.

Vanished. Never came back.

How could I dismiss acupuncture after that one success? But on the whole, the acupuncturist and I agreed he had probably accomplished as much as could be done at the time, although he recommended that I come in for an occasional "tune-up."

Two years later, I was back for a fresh series of treatments that I hoped would relax some facial muscles that were becoming increasingly rigid. I had some success. It still isn't easy, but now it's easier for me to use the telephone. During one of those sessions the acupuncturist told me about a successful stroke treatment that was now available in San Francisco if given immediately (a week or two after the stroke). He said the San Francisco acupuncturists were using an extremely specialized procedure, one that had not been included in his training in China.

In April, 2000, I found a reference on the Internet to America's growing interest in acupuncture. The Center for Integrative Health, Medicine, and Research in Santa Monica, California, announced a pilot research study at Emperor's College on the efficacy of this traditional three-thousand-year-old treatment for stroke rehabilitation. The planned pilot study will include sixty people who will undergo stroke rehabilitation at Daniel Freeman Rehabilitation Center associated with the University of Southern California, the University of California at Los Angeles's Arthur Ashe Center, the Los Angeles Free Clinic, Cedars-Sinai Hospital, and Daniel Freeman Hospitals.

Sixty people in a pilot project.

It will be many years before the information they gather, write up, and send out to be peer-reviewed, before it can be published, will be available for the rest of us.

Another report. This from a young man, horrified by his father's massive stroke, who is currently traveling around the world to see how people in other parts of the planet treat strokes.

In August, 2000, he visited China and sent this report on acupuncture to the stroke chat-room:

> *" How many million survivors currently live in China right now?" I asked Dr. Kong Lingzhi of the Ministry of Health.*
>
> *"Approximately 6 million," she responds.*
>
> *"And how many new cases of stroke are there per year?" I asked, leaning forward in my seat.*
>
> *"1.2 million."*

"One-point-two million?" I repeat... thinking, "hell, that's the entire population of Indianapolis, where I was born."

> *"How many people in China die every year from stroke?"*

35

"Eight hundred thousand to one million."

For a country with 1.2 billion people, China has a problem on its hands not only with stroke, but also with health care in general.

After meeting with Dr. Li Ying Cue of the Peking Union Hospital, I am under the impression that the Chinese population puts more of their trust in traditional Chinese medicine than in Western medicine.
With thousands of years of practice and improvements, Chinese medicine has made herbal medicines and acupuncture the treatment of choice for stabilizing the outcome of a stroke.

The young man concludes:

Because there is a huge rehabilitation deficit within the Chinese medical establishment, herbal medicines such as Dan Shen Co (a glucose), and Ge Gen Sum Chuan Quong Qin (used for microcirculation and blood vessel expansion) are used along with acupuncture in the later stages of stroke treatment. Both herbs and acupuncture have resulted in numerous and consistent success stories.

One point two million strokes a year! Six million survivors. The odds seem to be better in China. Clearly, acupuncture must be helpful in stroke rehabilitation because this treatment has survived for thousands of years. If a treatment doesn't work, it doesn't last very long. It will be interesting to see the results of the Santa Monica study.

4

I DISCOVER THE WORLD OF HYPERBARIC MEDICINE

Before my daughter sent me a book on heart problems she thought might interest me, I'd never heard of hyperbaric oxygen. Imagine my excitement when one of the chapters described strokes and hyperbaric oxygen, and new treatments that were in the works.

A new stroke treatment called "hyperbaric oxygen?"

Was I interested? You bet I was!

Amazon.com listed only one title with the words "hyperbaric oxygen." It was a paperback published by an alternative medicine press. *Hyperbaric Oxygen Therapy, using HBO Therapy to Increase Circulation, Repair Damaged Tissue, Fight Infection, Save Limbs and Relieve Pain,* by Neubauer and Walker. I ordered it, although when I saw that the book had been published by an alternative press, I'll admit I was a bit skeptical. When it arrived, however, I knew this was no flaky piece of New Age hocus-pocus.

Dr. Edward Teller, a world-famous nuclear physicist, and one of the scientists who masterminded the hydrogen bomb, had written the preface. After WWII, Dr. Teller had been the Director of Lawrence Livermore National Laboratory and was now an emeritus professor at several major universities. If a highly respected scientist with a background like Dr.

Teller's says the science is accurate, I knew I could trust the information. I was confident that he understood the basic theory underlying this new treatment called hyperbaric oxygen.

Dr. Teller had written:

> *This is founded on good science... I am recovering from a stroke caused by a clot that blocked blood flow to the brain ... There is a strong possibility that my healing will be accelerated by oxygen diffusing from some nearby capillary that hasn't been affected by the stroke... Possibly the most important applications (of hyperbaric oxygen) have been in the recovery of patients from stroke, multiple sclerosis, coma, and other damaged-nerve problems.*

Using the words "hyperbaric oxygen" as my new tool for finding stroke information, I looked up Dr. Richard Neubauer, co-author of the book I'd just received, and read:

> *Human beings can survive without food for weeks, and without water for days—but only minutes without oxygen. Oxygen is the basis of life...It can mean the difference between life and death, coma and mental alertness, paralysis and movement, illness and health. "*
>
> Richard A. Neubauer, M.D., Medical Director, Ocean Hyperbaric Center, Fort Lauderdale-by-the-Sea

Oxygen! Of course!

I felt as if I were one of those cartoon characters who has a brilliant insight and the cartoonist draws a bulb lighting up in his head.

When I read, "Oxygen under pressure can be forced into the fluid that feeds those hypoxic cells and dormant neurons return to normal activity," I felt like perhaps there was hope for me.

"Electricity can once again bridge the gaps between...neurons."

Your brain works!

Oxygen! It's so obvious. If a brain cell is dying because it isn't getting enough oxygen, GIVE THE BRAIN MORE OXYGEN.

But why had Neubauer and Walker published their book in an "alternative" press? Surely, oxygen is not "alternative" medicine?   Ridiculous. I'd been breathing it all my life.

Thanks to Dr. Neubauer, I learned for the first time what had actually been happening inside my head while I was having the stroke.

> *Stroke is caused by a sudden loss of blood and oxygen to a specific area of the brain, which kills off a central core of brain cells. With the death of these cells and the swelling caused by the original injury, blood and oxygen are further isolated from the surrounding cells, which then swell in a repeating cycle like the spreading ripples in a pond when you toss a stone in the water. This is the ischemic penumbra. It is these surrounding cells rather than the destroyed central core which causes 85 percent of the stroke patient's disability.*

Why isn't it standard practice, I wondered, to give oxygen to a patient having a stroke? We have billions of brain cells—somewhere between ten billion and one hundred billion. With those numbers, is it any wonder that the wiring inside our head sometimes breaks down? When that happens, isn't it logical to bring in an emergency supply of oxygen?

The Ischemic Penumbra and the Damage It Causes

Dr. Neubauer called the injured area an *ischemic penumbra*. This was new to me. No one on the medical staff at the hospital had said anything about an ischemic penumbra. Neither my primary-care doctor nor any of the stroke sites I'd found on the Internet had said or written anything about brain swelling or the development of an ischemic penumbra. I'd seen nothing that explained the devastating secondary damage. Nothing that told me why strokes are the leading cause of crippling disabilities.

As I write this several years later, I still don't find the words "pressurized oxygen," "ischemic penumbra," or "oxygen" on any university, government, or medical website offering general stroke information to the public. Why not? All the authorities agree that brain cells die without oxygen.

I know the damage had been progressive. I remembered how easily I had been able to use my right hand that morning, before I checked into the hospital. Holding a glass of orange juice had been no problem. Speaking had been effortless. All these problems had developed in the days following my stroke.

That was the moment when I realized that my frightening, unsteady balance and awkward limp, my stiff, sagging mouth, and clumsy right hand that can no longer write were caused by secondary swelling *that could have been prevented.*

This was a stunning piece of news.

Now that I had the magical words "hyperbaric oxygen" to use as my Open Sesame, the world of "strokes" opened up for me. I quickly found many information sites. Dr. David Steenblock, the Director of the Health Restoration Center in Mission Viejo, California, said in an address he'd given to the World Future Conference, May, 1996:

> *Approximately 700,000 persons suffer a stroke each year in the United States. Of these, 70 percent will suffer the type of stroke that is treatable by thrombolitic agents, but only a small percent of stroke victims will be able to get to a hospital during that short window of opportunity.*

He was describing the kind of stroke I'd had and the three-hour restriction that meant the emergency room doctor couldn't give me tPA, the only stroke treatment available.

Steenblock went on to say:

> *Currently there are more than four million people living with the after-effects of stroke disabilities. If you can get oxygen to the brain within the first 24 hours of a stroke, you can stop most of the injury and eliminate 70–80 percent of the damage.*

Four million victims? And seventy or eighty percent of their crippling disabilities could have been prevented?

At last! An explanation for why new problems had appeared each day while my "minor" stroke was stabilizing. Day by day, during that week in the hospital, new capillaries in my brain had been squeezed, disabling more and more brain cells.

But I didn't understand why my crippling disabilities weren't going away until I found this gem:

> More than thirty years ago, researchers who were studying "stroke" damaged the brain of a baboon to measure the flow of electricity in a living brain. They discovered that neurons in the injured area became totally non-functional when the blood-flow was reduced to 15 percent of normal, but those non-functioning cells could be revived. Later, when they examined sections of the damaged brain, they found "an ischemic marginal zone surrounding a central core," and named this chronically swollen area of living but dormant cells the "ischemic penumbra."
>
> Over the years, many scientists have duplicated these experiments, measuring the changes that occur when a brain's blood supply is blocked. Brain cells, they have learned, don't actually die until the level of blood-flow is reduced to as little as 10 percent of normal.

So the capillaries that swell while a stroke is developing don't have room for enough oxygen-carrying blood to reach dormant, living cells, and they remain swollen for years and years because they are getting some oxygen, but still not getting enough to be able to function normally. This explains why, when an area in the brain swells, the swelling doesn't just fade away in the same way swelling disappears after a broken bone is healed.

And oxygen would have prevented much of the swelling!

I was appalled.

Outraged.

Furious.

I know that oxygen at normal atmospheric pressure was available in our small community hospital, but I wasn't given any. Nor were any of the other stroke victims given oxygen—other men and women who were treated for strokes in our local community hospital. Was Dr. Steenblock saying that our small-town doctor had condemned each of us to struggle for the rest of our lives against these frustrating handicaps because *he didn't know enough to give oxygen to a stroke patient?*

Later, I learned Dr. Steenblock wasn't writing about oxygen at room pressures. He'd been describing pressurized oxygen that can be forced into the plasma.

But I can't help wondering...

Clearly my stroke damage had been progressive. Another new, crippling disability had appeared each day during that first week. If I had been given oxygen while my brain was under attack, wouldn't it have protected my still-normal capillaries? I later learned, and you will find in Chapter 8, that ordinary hospital oxygen at one atmosphere (14.7 p.s.i.) pressure is recommended for acute stroke treatment by the neurosurgeon K. K. Jain. But administering oxygen to a patient having an acute stroke is officially discouraged by the AMA, as I note in Chapter 6.

Every medical report I've found since I've been researching strokes has called "stroke" a hypoxic (oxygen-starvation) condition, but when I returned to the American Stroke Association's stroke treatment protocol posted on the Internet in 1997, I realized the emergency room doctor on duty in our local hospital had actually been following what the AMA says is the "Treatment of Choice." *Watch and wait until the patient has stabilized. Then talk to their loved ones about nursing homes and eventual therapy.*

In other words, our local doctor had followed accepted conventional medical advice. Leave the patient alone. Let the stroke fully develop. Don't bother trying to do anything to prevent or reduce the damage.

How can a respected, publicly funded organization like the American Heart Association advise any physician to *"Just watch and wait while devastating secondary damage develops,"* when there is a treatment that can limit or even prevent most of the damage? What has happened to medicine's Hippocratic Oath: DO NO HARM?

At that moment, this book was born.

Example of an Off-Label Post-Stroke Treatment

At this point I'd like to share an exciting story I found on the Hyperbaric Chat Line, March 1, 2001.

My husband had a massive brain aneurysm (bleed) in 1997, lay in one facility for almost 6 hours with little treatment before we could get him airflighted out. Then brain surgery and coma for almost 6 months. They told us he had bled too long — then, that if he lived, he would never wake up, that he would be a vegetable for the rest of his life.

He was away from the house another 6 months in 5 different rehab hospitals. They told us he would be in a wheelchair all his life and never talk or be able to be fed without a tube. "Nursing home" they all screamed. Family screamed, "Not in his lifetime."

I gave him acupuncture treatments and he walked. I started him back in the gym. I gave him nutritional supplements. I gave him chiropractic. I gave him ozone treatments. I gave him massage. You name it and if there was any chance it might help him, somehow we got it for him.

Bill was only 55 years old and we felt that if God had wanted him, he had that first 6 hours to take him when he received so little treatment, and yet he didn't. Bill had literally defied all the odds. His bleed could not have been in a worse area. Deep in the brain— left frontal lobe basal ganglia area. He had no short or long term memory and virtually no retention. He was incontinent, drooled constantly, dragged his right leg and was very bent over with his posture. He developed a massive dvt in right leg while in coma and we had to place a greenfield filter in stomach area to stop it from killing him should it move. He developed a blood pressure problem (never had before) and atrial fibrillation. He had to have a pacemaker. You name it, we have survived it. All these things helped.

But the one thing that we had been desperately trying to get for him from the moment he came out of surgery was HBOT (hyperbaric oxygen treatment). We did our research and that was the one thing we came up with. We talked to doctors here and in several different countries.

But, I did not get that accomplished until Aug, 2000—3 years post stroke. Bill literally "woke up" in the chamber after the 8th session. He became conversational. He stopped dragging his foot and leg almost completely. He stood more erect. The drooling ceased—except only a little when he is extremely tired. He rarely has a bathroom problem anymore, unless he just can't get get there in time.

He got 25 treatments. He has just completed 40 more. This time we noticed much improvement in memory retention and short term. Everyone was amazed at his further improvement. I have all this documented.

What I am trying to say is that of all the things I have done for Bill, HBOT is the thing that pushed him over the "hump."

I hope Bill's long journey back can be of help to you.

Allene Creacy

Actually, the story didn't end there. In the spring of 2001, this valiant lady mobilized the entire state of Texas. She asked the friends and relatives of people who have been successfully treated with hyperbaric oxygen to write, telephone, or visit their state representatives, telling the lawmakers about the improvements they'd either experienced or seen in others. Her campaign created such an overwhelmingly positive public response that the legislature passed Texas House Bill 1676, effective as of September 1, 2001, mandating that all health benefit insurance plans and health management organizations must accept requests for hyperbaric oxygen treatment for brain injuries or neurological damage. Texas is now a national leader. No longer can the US Food and Drug Administration, or any health maintenance organization doing business in Texas, casually brush aside a request for HBO treatment for a brain injury by calling it an "experimental, unapproved" treatment.

What Is HBO and How Does It Work?

There's oxygen in the air we breathe every day. Why isn't that good enough? This question is asked because we've been taught that it is the red blood corpuscles (hemoglobin), and only the red blood corpuscles, that carry oxygen, but the numbers change when air is compressed. At two times the sea level atmospheric pressure, or the equivalent of roughly thirty-three feet below sea level, the air holds twice as much oxygen, and this makes an enormous difference. That added oxygen can be carried in the plasma—the watery fluid that bathes every cell in our bodies.

Why is that useful? Imagine for a moment that the arteries and veins in our bodies are like pipes, and the pipes form a network of interconnected canals and ditches. The larger pipes, or arteries, are like freeways with smaller canals or tubes branching off into little tunnels that function like ordinary streets and alleys, and continue separating into capillaries that grow narrower and narrower until they resemble a multitude of narrow, twisting footpaths, one of which carries supplies to every cell in your body. Now, pretend that your red blood corpuscles are little red wagons and their task is to carry food and oxygen to each cell. The most oxygen that any red blood cell can hold is 1.34 milliliters. If every red blood cell is already carrying every bit of oxygen that it can hold, giving more oxygen to a patient would be useless.

But someone who is breathing 100 percent oxygen inside a chamber that has been pressurized to 1.5 atmospheres absolute (ATA), or the equivalent to breathing 150 percent oxygen at sea level, can be getting additional oxygen in the plasma, the fluid that carries the red blood cells. This means the oxygen-delivery system has been temporarily upgraded.

Now, instead of the normal parade of little red wagons piled high with oxygen, sugars, and other nutrients floating placidly along in your arteries, imagine there is a temporary obstruction somewhere in the pipeline. Maybe the problem is the result of an accident that has crushed a few fragile blood vessels, or one of the tubes may have been temporarily clogged by a bit of junk (clot) in the blood. The red blood corpuscles may have been blocked, but oxygen under pressure in the plasma can *still* slide past an obstruction, and this fluid or plasma can deliver oxygen to oxygen-starving or hypoxic tissues on the other side of the roadblock.

As Dr. Neubauer explained "stroke":

In tiny capillaries, those less than 1.5 mm in diameter, the red blood cells are squeezed into a column instead of randomly flowing in the plasma as they do in larger blood vessels. If the flow of blood slows in one of these very small blood vessels, the blood may thicken for a moment but plasma can still seep past the obstacle. When pressurized oxygen is forced into the plasma, the additional oxygen thins the fluid, stopping the formation of a penumbra.

Or as another hyperbaric oxygen specialist explains the theory of "pressurized oxygen":

It is common for physicians to argue that blood is saturated with oxygen when air is breathed at sea level, but one gram of hemoglobin can only transport 1.34 grams of oxygen...This explains why red blood cells are limited in the amount of oxygen they can deliver to tissue cells. Under hyperbaric conditions (at 1.5 ATA) the oxygen content of plasma is raised from 95mm Hg to over 2000mm Hg, thus increasing the available oxygen by 20-fold.

Injuries or conditions with swelling can restrict blood flow (ischemia) to the affected area of the body.

Severe tissue hypoxia (low oxygen levels) can be present, even when arterial tensions are normal if such circulatory factors as arterial occlusion, closure of the microcirculation and edema (water content in tissues) are present. When inflammation, edema or an invasion of metabolically active inflammatory cells are present, we can have hypoxia even when the blood flow per unit volume of tissue is increased.

5

HISTORY OF HYPERBARIC OXYGEN

The US Food and Drug Administration may call oxygen a "new" or "experimental" medical treatment, but it has been around a long time. And as several hyperbaric physicians have pointed out, oxygen is not an "alternative" medicine. It is the pills we swallow, the synthetic drugs and injections, the surgeries that slice into our bodies that are prescribed so freely today; those are "alternative" medicines. Oxygen is a natural substance, and therein lies its problem.

Oxygen cannot be patented because nobody can claim to have invented it. Therefore, no one can make a lot of money by using it to treat an injury or illness. Cynics have suggested that "profit" might be one of the reasons medical schools don't teach "oxygen." Another reason might be the astonishing and explosive growth and wide-ranging scope of medical research. Today's scientists can take a single cell apart, molecule by molecule, and analyze every biochemical interaction that goes on inside and outside of that cell. This ever-increasing knowledge has lured many scientists into a false sense of being able to control and manipulate every possible interaction between a cell and a synthetic drug. If one of these brilliant scientists doesn't succeed today, that's okay. Someone else, some day soon, will make the next breakthrough, and in the meantime, those widely advertised man-made pharmaceuticals currently being marketed under valuable patents are *VERY* profitable.

There are doctors who will laugh at you if you dare to ask about HBO. "Heavens no! That's just an 'old-fashioned' remedy." This true story was related on the Internet. The grieving parents of a baby who had been diagnosed as having cerebral palsy (brain-damaged at birth) asked their pediatrician if HBO could help their child, and the pediatrician just laughed. "Oh, no, ha ha ha. We don't do that any more!" Well, for his information, today many physicians *ARE* recommending HBO for brain-damaged children and are seeing and reporting impressive improvements in cognition, muscular control, and speech. (Dr. Neubauer's recent *Hyperbaric Oxygenation for Cerebral Palsy and the Brain-Injured Child*, Best Publishing Company.)

One hyperbaric physician trying to explain the resistance of today's older doctors to using oxygen said, "If they don't already know it, they think it's got to be quackery. Although," he added, "everyone knows that oxygen is the only treatment we have today for 'the bends' and non-healing wounds." Another said, "There's nothing as impossible as trying to convince someone that what he already knows is wrong."

What has led to this state of affairs?

Oxygen's healing qualities were recognized three hundred years ago by the British physician Henshaw, although it was another one hundred years before the element we call "oxygen" was even identified as one of the important elements of the air we breathe. In 1662, Henshaw, a man who was an ingenious inventor as well as an observant physician, designed and built a sort of hyperbaric chamber. His *domicillium* (tank) was connected to a large pair of organ bellows that were pumped to compress air. Dr. Henshaw used valves to increase the pressure when he was treating an acute disease, and decreased the pressure for chronic ailments. He advertised the benefits of his invention to the public, writing:

> *In times of good health this domicillium is proposed as a good expedient to help digestion, to promote insensible respiration, to facilitate breathing and expectoration and consequently, is of excellent use for prevention of most affectations of the lungs.*

In the 1770s, a Swedish apothecary, and at roughly the same time, the English chemist Priestly, identified and named the gaseous element we call "oxygen." Each man based his discovery on a law of physics (Henry's Law) that states: "The solubility of a gas is proportional to the pressure of the gas over the solution, provided that no chemical reaction occurs."

Pressurized air may have been useful and effective for treating Henshaw's patients, but his *domicillium* was unwieldy. In fact, it was so difficult to operate that the Dutch Academy of Sciences offered a prize in 1782 for an apparatus that would allow scientists to study the effect of varying oxygen pressures on living creatures. Unfortunately, there were no entries, so the prize was never awarded.

By the 1800s, pressurized oxygen had become fashionable throughout Europe. It was so popular in France that that nation became the world's leader in its use. Oxygen could, according to one advertisement:

> *Increase the circulation to the internal organs, improve cerebral blood flow and produce a feeling of well being as well as for treating various ailments. Such problems as tuberculosis, laryngitis, tracheitis and pertussis and unrelated diseases such as deafness, cholera, rickets, metrorhagia and conjunctivitis were included in the medical arsenal.*

Physicians of the era may not have understood exactly how or why oxygen was healing so many of their patients, and relieving painful chronic symptoms in others, but by the second half of the eighteenth century there were hyperbaric chambers in every major city in Europe. Many were touting the benefits of their "Pneumatic Institutes" as comparable to health spas.

Having a patient breath oxygen while undergoing surgery appeared to be extraordinarily helpful. In 1877, the French physician Fontaine built a mobile, fully-equipped hyperbaric operating room that allowed him to perform surgery in a hospital, a sanatorium, or even a private home. Fontaine claimed his patients recovered more quickly from nitrous oxide, the anesthetic of the day, that cyanosis and asphyxia were reduced, and vomiting was decreased. After twenty-seven successful operations, enthusiasm for his movable chamber was so great that a large surgical amphitheater, one that could hold 300 people, was designed. Unfortunately the huge unit was never built, but Fontaine had demonstrated the healing qualities of oxygen.

Sam Willian, M.D., a far-seeing English doctor, so appreciated oxygen in his practice that he published his observations in the British Medical Record, Oct. 31, 1885, pp 483–488:

> ...*The use of atmospheric air under different degrees of atmospheric pressure, in the treatment of disease, is one of the most important advances in modern medicine and when we consider the simplicity of the agent, the exact methods by which it can be applied, and the precision with which it can be regulated to the requirements of each individual, we are astonished that in England this method of treatment has been so little used.*
>
> *...there is no reason why enterprising practitioners who are not already too severely overworked, or who are too shiftless or indolent to incur the necessary preparations should long be without facilities with which to avail themselves of this potent therapeutic agent. It's use has long enough been surrendered to advertising quacks. It is time the regular profession rescued it from the smirch of charlantry which has, to some extent, heretofore attached to it.*

When I read this, I thought, "Truer words were never spoken. Some things never change."

In North America, the first hyperbaric chamber was opened in Oshawa, Ontario, back in 1869, and one was opened in New York a year later, advertised as treating "nervous and related disorders." Americans who needed the new therapy no longer had to travel to Europe.

Oxygen's Tarnished Reputation

The hyperbaric chamber that gave "oxygen" a bad name in America was opened in 1918 by Orval Cunningham, an anesthesiology professor at Kansas University Medical School in Kansas City. As an anesthesiologist, Cunningham had observed that heart disease and pneumonia patients living in the mountains did not recover as quickly or as easily as patients living at sea level. His imagination was triggered by this observation, and Cunningham received permission from the medical school to experimentally treat laboratory animals with oxygen, but his animal experiments were never completed. In 1918, the infamous Spanish influenza was sweeping the country, and people were begging Cunningham for hyperbaric air treatments.

He wrote up his results, saying he'd been remarkably successful when treating cyanotic and comatose patients. His claim sounds reasonable based on our knowledge of HBO. Cyanotic means a patient turns blue because his oxygen level is low, and comatose patients are frequently hypoxic. The survival rate of his patients was so high that people began flocking to him, asking him to treat their rheumatic fever, arthritis, syphilis, hypertension, diabetes, cancer, or whatever ailed them. Clearly oxygen wasn't a magical cure-all for everything. However, the multimillionaire Henry Timken, who recovered from a kidney infection and uremia after being desperately ill, was so impressed by the life-saving new oxygen treatment that he financed the construction of a luxurious, multi-story hyperbaric hospital in Cleveland, Ohio. This facility was operated by Cunningham.

The rest of the story is not so clear. The medical school at Kansas University asked Cunningham to resign because he was neither teaching nor practicing anesthesia, but Cunningham was also making a lot of money, and this apparently upset his peers. Some of the other physicians at the medical school called him a "quack," ignoring his high patient recovery rate. They accused him of administering "aero-therapy" without proper experimental data. Unfortunately, the American Medical Association took their side of the dispute, did a cursory investigation, and claimed there was no "evidence" to support his reports of successful treatments. Apparently, anecdotal evidence was ignored then, as it is today.

Cunningham, unfortunately, was so angered by what he called "persecution" that he refused to write up his results in the proper, "approved" fashion. The hospital flourished until the crash of '29, when patients could no longer afford the treatments. Cunningham's health was said to be failing, so he turned the hospital operations over to a young assistant. A year later the hospital closed. Cunningham's oxygen chamber, a steel sphere, was dismantled and turned into scrap metal during World War II.

Was this a failure of hyperbaric oxygen therapy to successfully treat so many sick, hurting people? Or a sad example of political pressures and professional jealousy? Of ignorance? The record doesn't say. But the story is widely circulated as a "failure" of HBO.

Even today, within the hyperbaric community there is a sharp division of opinion. Some doctors look at the facts—oxygen is essential to life, essential for healing to take place, and they want to offer the best medical treatment available to their patients. Others are afraid of being tarred by Cunningham's reputation—the so-called "quack" who refused to submit his results to a jury of his antagonistic peers. Some hyperbaric specialists choose to limit the use of oxygen to only those "safe" ailments that have already been approved by the powerful FDA. Oxygen is their "turf," and they want to protect it from any and all threats. As the editor of a hyperbaric newsletter says, "In science itself there are numerous barriers to free expression: territorial protection, strong economic and political interests, and rivalries that result in the suppression of new ideas."

Shakespeare expressed the same idea when he wrote, "The good that men do is oft interred with their bones. The evil lives on after them."

The Bends

Modern medical hyperbaric oxygen owes its existence to the industrial revolution of the 1800s, and most particularly to the inventions of high-capacity compressed air pumps and the diving bell. The diving bell meant men could work under water in *caissons,* or underwater chambers that were filled with compressed air and large enough to allow several men at a time to work on a construction project. Sometimes the workers were in the *caisson* for seven hours at a stretch, at an average depth of sixty-five feet. They didn't have any medical complaints while they were working, but as soon as they left the *caisson* they began to have dizzy spells or couldn't stop coughing. They were short of breath. Their joints ached or they had severe abdominal cramps. No one knew why, but the aches and pains seemed to go away when they were back at work in the *caisson*.

By 1854, the French physicians Pol and Watelle realized it was only those working in a compressed air environment who were having these mysterious new aches and pains, and that their symptoms were relieved when they were once again breathing pressurized air.

By the late 1800s, scientific instruments had been developed that were so sensitive that scientists could measure the effects of increasing or decreasing atmospheric pressures on the human body. The French physiologist Paul Bert published his findings in 1876. *Maladie de caisson,* as the ailment was termed, was caused by nitrogen bubbles forming in a worker's blood when he left the pressurized air too rapidly. Bert suggested a gradual reduction in pressure could dissolve the bubbles and additional oxygen could wash the nitrogen out.

In America, the disease began to show up in men who were working in large tanks filled with compressed air under the Hudson River while constructing the Holland Tunnel, and in workmen laying the footings for the Brooklyn Bridge. Americans called the disease "The Bends" because of the bent-over posture of the stricken workmen; they quickly discovered the Bends could be fatal. During the earliest construction phase, a quarter of the underwater workers died. Bert suggested that a man working in a compressed air environment should not be allowed to leave immediately after finishing his shift, but should go next to a relatively slow decompression chamber. The French physiologist's recommendation saved many lives. After the Americans tried his solution, the death rate dropped dramatically, and today is non-existent.

HBO and Decompression Sickness— How Does It Work?

The air we breathe every day is surprisingly heavy. The Naval Aerospace Medical Institute calls the atmosphere "an ocean of gases which extend from the Earth's surface to space," containing molecules that can be weighed and measured. At sea level, the air is made up roughly of 78 percent molecules of nitrogen, 21 percent molecules of oxygen and 1 percent of various other gases, weighing 14.7 pounds per square inch. When you climb a mountain or go up in a plane, the volume of air in your inner ear expands, making your ears "pop." Go scuba diving, where the atmosphere now includes the weight of the water over your head as well the weight of all those molecules of nitrogen and oxygen in the air, and you feel an increased pressure on your ears. Your eardrums are reacting to changes in the ambient pressure.

By definition, when you condense air, you are squeezing additional molecules of nitrogen and oxygen into the air you are compressing. This means a scuba diver breathing from a tank is inhaling more molecules of nitrogen and oxygen with each breath than he would at sea level. His body will use most of the added oxygen, so those added oxygen molecules are no problem for the diver's body.

On the other hand, nitrogen is an inert gas, one not used by the body. At sea level, nitrogen just floats around in the blood until it is exhaled. But at added pressure, those added nitrogen molecules begin to work their way into body cavities and tissues—the muscles, joints, nerves, or spinal fluid. That still doesn't create a problem for the diver unless he comes back to the surface too quickly. He must give the nitrogen molecules time to leave the various tissues or wherever they have temporarily been absorbed.

Something odd happens to nitrogen when the atmospheric pressure is changed. The example usually given is that of an unopened bottle of soda water. When you hold it up to the light, the soda looks exactly like water. You can't see any bubbles. But open the bottle and you'll hear a swoosh of released gas. Now you do see bubbles. As you watch, you'll notice more bubbles appearing and floating up to the surface. Put a stopper back on the bottle and the bubbles stop.

In this example, you've been watching bubbles of carbon dioxide, but nitrogen acts the same way. High pressure flows to low pressure. When you took the cap off, you released, or lowered, the pressure inside the bottle. With the ambient pressure lowered, the carbon dioxide that had been dissolved in the beverage turned back into gas-filled bubbles. The bubbles were lighter than the beverage they'd been dissolved in, so they floated up to the surface and into the air.

Essentially, that's what happens in a diver's body. When the ambient pressure is increased, that 79 percent nitrogen in the air the diver has been breathing dissolves into his blood and is carried throughout his body. It's no problem as long as the diver remains at depth, but divers don't stay forever underwater. They have to return to sea level and that's when nitrogen gas bubbles begin to come out of solution. As the diver comes up and the weight of the water or the pressure on his body is decreased, some nitrogen molecules in the blood start to come out of solution as gas bubbles. The longer a diver stays down, the more nitrogen gas will be absorbed in his body tissues. It's not a problem if he rises slowly enough for all the gas to be exhaled through his lungs during respiration, but when the ambient pressure is decreased too fast, the bubbles can expand in his joints, muscles, or tissue (brain or spinal column). It isn't the presence of nitrogen that does the damage. It's the size of the bubbles, where they are, and the body's ability to exhale them before they are trapped in the tissues of the body. The longer a diver has been under increased ambient pressure, the more nitrogen that has been absorbed into body tissues. As Dr. Bert found, decompression sickness is a result of both the *depth* of the dive and the *time* spent at depth.

What does all this have to do with strokes and hyperbaric medicine? Let me quote from an article by Stephen A. Pulley, Director of Emergency Medicine at Philadelphia College, and his associates that was posted on *Medicine*'s site for decompression sickness:

The basic theory behind hyperbaric therapy is to first repressurize the patient to a depth where the bubbles from nitrogen or air are redissolved into the body tissues and fluids. Then, by breathing intermittently higher concentrations of oxygen, a larger diffusion gradient is established. The patient is brought slowly back to surface atmospheric pressure. This allows gases to diffuse gradually out of the lungs and body...

HBO typically results in significant improvement in severe neurological DCS if it is identified and the patient transported to a hyperbaric facility rapidly...

An important issue is transport of the patient to the closest hyperbaric facility. This frequently is accomplished by land transport, however occasionally air transport is required. Helicopter transport necessitates the pilot maintaining altitude at less than 1000 feet. Fixed-wing transport should be limited to aircraft that can maintain cabin pressure at surface 1 ATA.

Dr. Pulley's third paragraph includes another important aspect of the way that *dysbarism,* or too-rapid atmospheric changes, either down or up in pressure, affects people. Aviators, too, can be attacked and even crippled by decompression sickness.

Bert and other French scientists were correct when they warned that the length of time a man worked inside a compressed-air-filled *caisson* and how quickly he left the tank were correlated. The aches, pains, and nausea were particularly noticeable when the change was made too quickly because decompression sickness is the result of large bubbles of excess nitrogen expanding in body tissues. It was the size of the bubbles that was important because when a bubble exits tissue, it must first enter a tiny capillary to get into a vein that is returning blood to the lungs to pick up fresh oxygen. The larger and more numerous the nitrogen bubbles, the greater the possibility they will cause symptoms. Neurological symptoms are more common in overweight people because nitrogen is attracted to fat and dissolves 5.3 times faster into fat than in blood. This results in the molecules' rapid movement into the fatty myelin sheaths that surround and protect nerves. As the diver rises, the nitrogen dissolves out of these nerve sheaths, but the bubbles can grow larger. Sometimes the growing cluster of molecules get stuck in a tiny capillary, compressing the nerve cells.

When a bubble gets trapped in nerve tissue, it can set off chemical reactions that are called "inflammatory response." An inflammatory response contains protein factors that can damage the blood vessel and affect blood clotting. MRIs are useful for imaging and treating the neurological aspects of decompression sickness.

Sound like the description of a stroke? A clot or bubble, creating an expanding "inflammatory response."

I thought so when I began to read and study about HBOT.

The only effective treatment for decompression sickness is time spent in a recompression chamber, the sooner the better. Recompression squeezes the nitrogen bubbles, causing them to go back into solution, thus eliminating bubbles. Any delay in hyperbaric treatment can leave a diver with permanent aches, pains, or even paralysis. The experts recommend prompt treatment in a hyperbaric chamber even when the pain seems to have vanished before the patient reaches the facility because Doppler imaging has revealed the presence of small, harmless nitrogen bubbles in a diver's blood for many hours after a diver has returned to sea level.

One unintended result of Bert's research was the discovery that too much oxygen, like too much of any substance, could be dangerous. It wasn't until 1936 that Dr. Albert Behnke reported to the medical world that oxygen safety was a matter of depth (increased ambient pressure), how long the person was breathing 100% oxygen, and his physical activity. As explained in *Scuba Diving Explained,* L. Martin, M.D., 1997, oxygen poisoning is not a problem for recreational scuba divers because scuba diving is limited to a depth of 130 feet on air.

Oxygen Today

Dangerous or not, oxygen was much too useful to be ignored by the medical profession. As early as 1908, the British Navy developed Haldane's Tables, a set of depth levels and length of time that could be safely spent by a man breathing compressed air. Based on Haldane's theory, the U.S. Navy developed a similar set of Decompression Tables in 1915 to combat decompression sickness because the world's engineers were still designing bridges and water was still trickling into tunnels and mines. Newly located undersea oil fields couldn't be pumped without offshore drilling platforms. The world's navies had new jobs for their divers. Jet planes meant that pilots in partially-pressurized planes risked nitrogen bubbles in their blood. NASA needed oxygen for pilots and for astronauts before they could explore space.

How Does The Oxygen Controversy Affect "Stroke" Medicine?

In 1965, Ingevar and Lassen were the first physicians to describe the positive results of treating stroke patients with oxygen. In that same year, the neurologist Illingworth published his results after giving 100 percent oxygen at a pressure of 1.5 atmospheres absolute to four stroke patients. Illingworth reported that three of his patients showed great improvement, but the fourth, who was already severely brain-damaged and comatose, died. When I heard these three-out-of-four odds, I thought, "They are better than we get today, and that was almost forty years ago." Why is oxygen still controversial in the medical world if this is the case?

What does it take to convince some people?

By 1980, Drs. Neubauer and End had treated 122 stroke patients with pressurized oxygen, measured their improvements with EEG and CT scans, and reported their results in a well-known medical journal:

Neubauer, R.A., End, E., Hyperbaric oxygenation as an adjunct therapy in strokes due to thrombosis. A review of 122 patients. Stroke ll(3), May-Jun 1980.

Dr. Neubauer has continued to report on successfully treated stroke patients. In a letter published in *Lancet*, June 29, 1991, he explains oxygen's role during an acute stroke:

> *Hyperbaric oxygen (HBOT) efficiently increases the diffusional driving force of oxygen, thereby increasing tissue oxygen availability. This overcomes ischemic/hypoxia and so reduces cerebral edema, restores integrity to the blood-brain barrier and cell membranes, neutralizes toxic amines, promotes phagocytosis, scavenges free radicals, stimulates angiogenesis and reactivates idling neurons...*
>
> *Earlier intervention rendered a more pronounced effect on stopping or limiting the ischemic cascade associated with the multiple biochemical actions that take place as the body's defense against hypoxia. Our interpretation is that after the acute ischemic incident, a settling process is mediated with the establishment of the ischemic penumbra.*

In another paper Dr. Neubauer explains "stroke" in this way:

> *In tiny capillaries, those less than 1.5 mm in diameter, the red blood cells are squeezed into a column instead of randomly flowing in plasma as they do in larger blood vessels. If the flow of blood slows in one of these very small blood vessels, the blood may thicken for a moment but plasma can still seep past the obstacle. When pressurized oxygen is forced into the plasma, the additional oxygen thins the fluid,*

stopping the formation of a penumbra.

To obtain a collection of similar current reports, refer to Dr. Steenblock's user-friendly hyperbaric website (www.strokedoctor.com).

After reading those reports, I felt a twinge of hope. Perhaps I had a bunch of sleeping cells inside my head. Could they really be awakened?

I went back to Dr. Neubauer's book and found:

> *There are only about 400 hyperbaric oxygen facilities in all of the United States and less than 2 percent of those hyperbaric chambers are used for neurological applications.*

Only four hundred HBO chambers throughout our entire nation, and only two percent of those chambers are used to treat stroke victims. When stroke symptoms are so similar to those seen in decompression sickness and HBO is *the* approved therapy, why is it used so infrequently for strokes? Doctors agree that brain cells must have oxygen or die. They've had that information for the last forty years. That bit of information stopped me in my tracks.

Much later, I was saddened to learn that a few hyperbaric chamber operators are *still* refusing to treat children with cerebral palsy or anyone who has received a traumatic brain injury (head wound, i.e., a car crash victim), even when a hyperbaric chamber is available. And I was shocked to learn that the US Food and Drug Administration, despite Texas Bill 1676, *still* says HBOT is an "experimental and unapproved" treatment for nerve and brain injuries. It is this attitude that has allowed so many ostrich-like physicians and tight-fisted HMOs to continue denying or casually ignoring HBO's benefits.

One physician on the HBO-list@hyperbaric.com, 21 April 2000, wrote:

> *Insurance denial is not necessarily a denial of necessity, just a refusal to pay for it. I believe a lot of insurance companies are afraid of the flood gates that would open if they accept HBOT for all the maladies it would help.*

I think those denials are appalling and sad. They are causing so much unnecessary pain and suffering.

Role of Government in Stroke Medicine

Many hospitals and medical facilities have said HBO is too inconvenient to administer and too expensive. They state that it requires trained personnel. Pills are easier and more efficient. Yet, those same hospitals advertise expensive new imaging equipment they have just purchased; their expensive new equipment requires highly trained personnel. And the pills they so readily prescribe are costly and not nearly as effective as oxygen. If private hospitals continue to tell us they can't afford to offer hyperbaric oxygen facilities to patients, the federal government would actually *SAVE* money by installing a hyperbaric oxygen chamber in every hospital in America.

It's not an unreasonable idea.

Making HBO available throughout the nation wouldn't increase the amount of dollars the government is already spending on health care. It would be a simple matter of transferring funds from one federally funded medical account to another, or of "robbing Peter to pay Paul." The latest figures from the National Stroke Association report that we're already spending 43 billion dollars a year for stroke treatment. The National Institutes of Health's website figures, quoted from *The Stroke/Brain Attack Reporter's Handbook,* published by the National Stroke Association, show the government is currently spending $28 billion a year for stroke care and therapy. The NIH estimates indirect costs to the government from lost wages and other factors is roughly $15 billion per year. In other words, the U.S. dollars we're already spending on strokes through Medicaid and Medicare would cover the cost of making HBO available to every person in the United States of America.

I'm not talking about just "stroke" damage and therapy. Many industrial and developing countries around the world are routinely using HBO to treat a wide range of conditions, illnesses, and injuries.

Who Already Uses HBO in the United States?

The Armed Forces know HBO is useful and they use it extensively. The U.S. Air Force School of Aerospace Medicine, the leading agent for the Department of Defense Hyperbaric Medicine program, which has been functioning since 1984, calls its hyperbaric oxygen program "well established in the treatment of many chronic diseases...associated with decompression illnesses and the resolution of physical ailments involving nitrogen gas in high altitude mishaps, as well as diving."

According to the U.S. Naval Flight Surgeon's manual:

> *The most frequently encountered hazard in aviation history is hypoxia. Records of early balloon and aircraft flights describe tragedies resulting from hypoxia, since even these primitive machines had a higher operational ceiling than the men aboard them.*
>
> *Hypoxia was a serious aviation problem in both World Wars and remains a potential threat in today's military aviation...Yet hypoxia continues to occur, and the flight surgeon should be well informed concerning this problem.*
>
> *...One of the earliest effects of hypoxia is impairment of judgment. Therefore even if the early symptoms are noted, an aviator may disregard them and often does, or he may take corrective action which is actually hazardous, such as disconnecting himself from his only oxygen supply. Finally, at high altitudes hypoxia may cause unconsciousness as the first symptom.*

At an Aerospace Medical Association meeting, Dr. James Wright, from the Davis Hyperbaric Laboratory, stated, "trauma, large blood loss, and advances in science and technology have called attention to the potential uses of a portable HBO machine for treating wounds in the battlefield."

The Air Force operates a massive clinical hyperbaric facility at Travis Air Force Base in California and one at Wright-Patterson Air Force Base,

Ohio. The Navy has a small unit on every ship and maintains large, land-based hyperbaric facilities in Pensacola, Florida, and Singapore, and is currently building a three-story, state-of-the-art hyperbaric medical facility at Portsmouth Naval Hospital in Virginia.

The Veteran's Administration at Long Beach, California, uses HBO for treating veterans, although treatment is limited to such FDA-approved disabilities as bone infections and those needing orthopedic (bone repair) healing or oral surgery.

The Department of Hyperbaric Medicine at the Wright-Patterson Air Force Base describes their oxygen program as:

> *Quality health care for all patients enrolled in standard treatment and for those who require emergency treatment...*
>
> *The hyperbaric medicine department also acts as a worldwide referral center for the military patient who sustains battlefield trauma resulting in soft tissue injury, infection, compromised circulation, or crush injury. HBOT can be especially useful in limiting the extent of injury and allowing earlier repair for reconstruction.*

Nothing in Wright-Patterson's patient brochure or that of any other facility maintained by the Armed Forces describes HBO as an "unproved, experimental" therapy.

Furthermore, the Armed Forces teach hyperbaric medicine. They maintain an active Hyperbaric Medicine program at the Uniformed Services

University of Health Sciences, allowing servicemen and women to earn a degree in HBO Medical Specialization. It is reassuring to know that the men and women in the Armed Forces have access to the best available medical care. We gladly pay for these life-saving facilities because we want our sons and daughters to receive the best care possible, but what about their parents, their brothers and sisters in civilian life? What about the aging taxpayers whose taxes built these HBO facilities?

I believe the Armed Forces have a moral obligation to refute the scornful sneers of a few civilian medics—uninformed doctors who still insist on calling oxygen an "outdated, outmoded treatment," and dismissing every reported success story as merely "anecdotal." I have noticed that many of the hyperbaric specialists posting messages on today's Internet are former Armed Services personnel who have either learned the technology, seen the results for themselves, or have been successfully treated.

A wealth of information has now been posted on the Internet—Google listed more than 1,560,000 citations containing the key words "oxygen treatment," "traumatic brain injury," "stroke," "cerebral edema," "near hanging," and "near drowning." The problems are there and so are the solutions, although they are not available to the rest of us. Why are only forty-six medical schools throughout the entire United States teaching "oxygen"?

Who Is Using HBO in the Academic World?

Among the first thirty HBO listings I found on the Internet were Duke University, Johns-Hopkins, and the University of California at Los Angeles, although the UCLA listing specified only "wound healing." Duke University's website says they have been operating a hyperbaric research and treatment program since 1963 and expanded their facility in 1978. The hyperbaric department has produced over a thousand research publications. Duke is one of the many universities that have rigorously examined hyperbaric oxygen and found that it does work.

The Next Obstacle

Now that we've established the fact that oxygen is recognized as a safe, natural, medically useful tool, let's look at the next obstacle. How much does a hyperbaric oxygen facility cost? How expensive would it be to equip every hospital in America with an HBO chamber and trained personnel?

In terms of today's sophisticated, high-tech medical equipment, an HBO facility is actually just a chamber that can withstand high pressure. It is merely a large tank to store compressed gases and a bunch of inlet and outlet pipes, control valves, and gauges in order to deliver the gas to a patient. The technology is simple and might be compared to that of the tank-truck carrying gases under pressure on our highways.

Currently, chambers range from approximately eighty thousand dollars for a single patient unit to multiplace chambers that can hold four, six, or as many as twelve people who can be treated at the same time. The multiplace units are currently advertised in the low hundreds of thousands of dollars, but it's reasonable to assume the cost would come down if every hospital bought one.

A hyperbaric oxygen chamber does require trained operators because oxygen can be a fire hazard unless it is carefully controlled. The same is true of all of the expensive diagnostic, imaging, and treatment equipment in a modern hospital that must be carefully installed. Every such instrument requires well-trained people. Hospitals pride themselves on the imaging and radiation equipment they've purchased for treating cancer, saying, "If you can't see it, you can't treat it." The same is true for a person having a stroke.

Today, a physician *CAN* see what is happening while a brain is under attack by using sophisticated new MRI or SPECT equipment. If they can see it, they ought to be willing to treat it. Unfortunately, too many physicians are still ignoring the healing qualities of pressurized oxygen because the US Food and Drug Administration continues to call oxygen an "unproven," "experimental" drug.

This is nonsense! Oxygen is neither outdated, unproven, nor untested. We have all been breathing it all our lives. Just try living an hour or so without it.

Something has to change.

6

CURIOUSER AND CURIOUSER

One evening as I was skimming the evening paper and listening to the evening news, I half heard Dan Rather say on TV, "America is only thirty-seventh in the world in terms of health care." I almost jumped out of my chair. Had Dan Rather really said health care in the United States was ranked so low that it was only thirty-seventh *in the whole world?* How could this be true? We are constantly being told that we are "the strongest, richest, luckiest people on the planet, that the health care we get in the United States is the most advanced, the finest..."

The next morning I looked up the World Health Organization on the Internet. And there it was.

The U.S. spends more dollars on health care in terms of gross national product than any other country in the world, but they rank 37th in survival rates out of a total of 191 countries. France was number one and Italy had the second best health care record in the world.

Although significant progress has been achieved in past decades, virtually all countries are underutilizing the resources that are available to them. This leads to large numbers of preventable deaths and disabilities; unnecessary suffering, injustice, inequality, and denial of an individual's basic right to health.

WHO 2000 Press Release

Other modern industrial nations do spend less money per person on health care than we do, but they get "more bang for their buck." If we're so clever, why aren't we getting more for our money?

Searching the Internet for answers, I found Alice in Wonderland's words "curiouser and curiouser" were oddly appropriate. The medical condition "stroke" appeared to exist in two very separate universes.

Both worlds agreed on one basic fact:

> *The body can protect itself from starvation by storing up glucose as fat, but the brain has no way to store an emergency supply of oxygen...brain cells die when their oxygen is cut off.*

But I found an enormous gap between the conventional American medical universe of pills and the world of oxygen therapy. The hyperbaric people said, "Quick! Give the brain oxygen. Those brain cells need it *right now!*" We can deliver it.

While the American world of pills was saying, "Er... uh...ahem...you have to realize...uh...that stroke is a very...er...uh...very complicated situation. We have created a wonderful new drug that can dissolve blood clots, and we're working on an even better one, but you people haven't been doing your part. If you don't get yourself to a hospital within the first three hours, well...we're sorry. Any stroke damage you are left with is all your fault."

They're working on a "newer and better drug"? One that can replace oxygen? Why would anyone spend research and development money on something as complicated and difficult to treat as a stroke when oxygen is already available?

Why not just use the real thing?

Doctors throughout the rest of the world have been using this simple technique to treat a multitude of hypoxic (oxygen-deprived) conditions. Take China, for example. With one-fifth of all the people in the world living in China, the national health care providers need to spend their money wisely. In 1998, the Chinese government was operating more than three thousand HBO facilities because Chinese doctors have found HBO to be useful and cost-effective for treating any oxygen-restricted or hypoxic condition. England lists some three hundred or more free-standing hyperbaric chambers, and says HBO is extremely helpful in slowing the devastation of multiple sclerosis. Every hospital in Japan has at least one hyperbaric chamber. Germany, Russia, and Cuba report the routine use of pressurized oxygen to treat a wide range of illnesses and injuries. I've recently seen stories from Argentina and South Africa describing their use of pressurized oxygen.

The World Health Organization is correct. We're spending tons of money on profitable, expensive new medical products, but we aren't getting our money's worth. Maybe we deserve our ranking of only thirty-seventh in the world in good health care.

Why are American doctors still ignoring HBO, a treatment the rest of the world finds safe and effective?

For centuries, medicine was a "trial-and-error" process. If one clever doctor found a remedy or procedure that had helped or cured one of his patients, he told other doctors, and they either used the new treatment or ignored it. If the new treatment failed, it was soon forgotten. When it worked, it quickly became standard practice because nothing succeeds like success.

Fortunately for me, the medical profession was not peer-review "hidebound" when ether was first discovered. Surgeries and amputations were performed without an anesthetic for most of human history, but when I was a child and my swollen and inflamed appendix was in danger of bursting, it was surgically removed while I was peacefully "asleep," and I recovered. No problem. It is true that even today, in spite of modern antibiotics and sterile surgical environments, people still occasionally die of appendicitis. Appendectomies aren't *always* one hundred percent successful, but my doctor knew the procedure usually worked, and he used it.

Not so today. "Anecdotal" medical reports are ignored *unless* the treatment is backed by a pharmaceutical company. It has become medically fashionable to ignore any treatment that has not been peer-reviewed and widely tested by other physicians in spite of a study *(N.Engl.J.Med.* 22 June 2000) comparing the results of anecdotal studies with the results of randomized, rigidly controlled scientific trials. The researchers were astonished to find almost no difference (less than .02 percent) in the results of each report. In other words, an "anecdotal" report of a treatment that worked was just as valid today as the results of a rigidly controlled, peer-reviewed scientific study. When a procedure works, it works. And a "peer review" doesn't necessarily mean an unbiased appraisal. Such a review can easily be slanted by asking only physicians who share your own set of beliefs and prejudices to look over the new information. This will almost guarantee that the fellow physicians you choose will agree with you that the "new" remedy is not worth considering.

It wasn't until the 1950s and an explosive mass of scientific breakthroughs that American medicine began to insist on these randomized, placebo-controlled, blind cross-over, peer-reviewed studies. Today's medical world has encouraged an attitude of hard-nosed, cynical skepticism. This mind set was probably established, in part, by tales of unscrupulous "snake oil salesmen," like those rascals in Mark Twain's *Huckleberry Finn* who literally "made" money by selling ordinary bottled Mississippi river water to gullible country folk as a cure-all for gout, morning sickness, scrofula, or whatever ailed you. And, in part, by what Linus Pauling and several other eminent scientists have called, "deliberate deceit on the part of a few."

The current vogue for skepticism is neither clear-sighted nor useful. Recently I was told that a neurologist in Oregon, when asked about HBO, replied, "I haven't seen any good science to validate the 'oxygen' theory." Clearly, he has never been oxygen-deprived. I'm sure any of the guys who have ever served aboard a submarine were ardent supporters of the "oxygen" theory.

UMs or Unprofitable Modalities

The key word here is "unprofitable." The code words UMs, or Unprofitable Modalities, represent those basic medications that are either ignored or actively rejected because they can't be patented, although they may be more effective, have fewer side effects, and provide a much better quality of life for a patient. This attitude is also true when the drug or treatment is so cheap or readily available that a pharmaceutical firm can't make a substantial profit by selling it.

The direction medicine is following has been observed with alarm and regret by some of today's leading medical authorities. A Harvard Medical School professor, physician, and former editor of the *New England Journal of Medicine* wrote in 1992:

> *Our health-care system, formerly a social service that was the responsibility of dedicated professionals and not-for-profit facilities, has become a vast, profit-oriented industry...Providers (of drugs) for the industry constantly strive to increase their profitability, but unlike other industries, their consumers have little control over the purchase and consumption of their products and services.*

Another long-time physician and former editor of the *NEJM* wrote in an editorial entitled, "Is Academic Medicine for Sale?":

> *Young physicians learn that for every problem there is a pill and the writer quoted the eminent immunologist Alan S. Levin who had complained of*

this unsettling financial emphasis in 1983, writing:
"In a recent sample issue of possibly the world's largest
and most prestigious medical journal there were 51
pages of scientific matter and 99 pages of industry
ads. Industry is setting the standard of medical
practice and has invaded the academic institutions:
as much as two-thirds of the research funding in most
major institutions comes directly or indirectly from
industry interests." Levin concluded by saying, "if you
don't think medicine is being taken over by industry...
read any of the so-called peer review journals and
you will realize they are dominated by industry."

Unfortunately for the public, medical journals depend on those profitable ads.

John Ely, Ph.D., an orthomolecular biologist and chair of radiation studies at the University of Washington, who has been studying CoEnzyme Q10 and stroke since 1972, says, "Unfortunately, a small number of the Unprofitable Modalities are essential nutrients without which a human cannot have a long or healthy life." He calls the rejection of CoQ10 and ascorbic acid "possibly the most lethal errors in modern medicine, because no cell or organ can function unless these essential nutrients are present." Ely names Linus Pauling of vitamin C fame, Wilfred and Evan Shute, who were early and vigorous proponents of vitamin E for healthy hearts, James Watson, who won a Nobel for describing the double helix structure of chromosomes, and several other, equally well-known medical researchers as being alarmed by "the current state of medicine as the sole judge of its own quality, and historically calloused in its slowness to eliminate long-held erroneous medical beliefs." Ely believes today's rejection of unprofitable drugs costs the U.S. more than a million early patient deaths per year and over one trillion dollars annually. Oxygen is frequently called an "unprofitable drug" because it is cheap and cannot be patented.

I believe today's doctors have thrown the baby out with the bath water, and that the World Health Organization is right. We *are* under-utilizing our resources.

How has this happened?

As my daughter Jane, the medical researcher, reminds me, "This gets to the question of what we know, how we know what we know, and how doctors know what they know."

In medical school a doctor must learn the name, location, and function of every bone, muscle, and organ in the human body. That's a daunting amount of information to stuff into the head of any young person. It's not surprising that if the required medical school curriculum has not included the science of "pressurized oxygen," our modern doctors honestly believe they are being "scientifically rigorous" when they ignore any treatment that has not been randomized, placebo-controlled, blind cross-over and peer-reviewed.

A new procedure can be scientifically valid and be overlooked because the doctor, or some member of the county medical board that oversees his work, isn't aware of an effective therapy. Thus, the benefits of the new procedure won't be offered to patients.

Patients are the losers in this instance.

Why?

Today's doctors, the kindly clinical physicians and specialists who care for us, have other major problems. First, they are deluged with information. Ely says millions of pages of recognized medical science research and clinical literature have been published during the past fifty years. Indeed, he writes, another forty million pages are published every ten years. Buried in those millions of pages could lie countless UMs that have been demonstrated to be better, safer, and more effective than the current standard Treatment of Choice.

Then, there is an ever-increasing flood of medical journals and a wealth of conferences. Additionally, today's insurance companies and health management organizations are demanding mountains of paperwork. Ely says, "In addition to the literature [and paperwork problems], there are constraints imposed by medical disciplinary boards that forbid departing from Treatment of Choice."

The simple truth is that today's doctors have too little time to just be doctors, but the biopharmaceutical giants have come to the rescue.

The drug companies have hired an army of salespeople called "detail men," and they send these men and women out on the road to "help" our overburdened doctors stay current. It's fact; doctors need to be told about the benefits of a salesman's latest products before they will prescribe it for a patient, or know what to say when a patient "asks his doctor," as we are constantly urged to do. These detail men and women are well educated. They know how to talk about medicine when they visit a doctor in her or his office.

During the visit, they sometimes offer an overworked physician a chance to "learn the latest" by getting away—attending a seminar at some glamorous vacation spot, organized and paid for by the salesman's firm, of course. The pharmaceutical companies want every doctor to understand the unique qualities of some miracle drug that the firm has spent ten million dollars to create, and the drug companies are also constantly haranguing a defenseless public to "just ask your doctor."

While the detail guy is describing his pills, he may just "happen" to mention some new, off-label use for one of his firm's products. In other words, he is actually suggesting that the doctor practice "anecdotal" medicine. In spite of their heated denials, many doctors *are* practicing *"anecdotal"* medicine today. When a drug or substance works, that's great. It's the way medical care has always advanced.

On Jan. 10, 2004, the *New York Times* printed the following by Dan Shapiro, M.D., of the University of Arizona, who wrote that there is a growing concern in the medical world over the influence of the pharmaceutical industry on doctors:

> ...Meredith Rosenthal of the Harvard School of Public Health reported in the New England Journal of Medicine that the industry spends roughly 15.7 billion annually marketing medications, with 4.8 billion dedicated to detailing individual physicians, or roughly $6,000 to $11,000 a doctor a year.

Studies indicate that most physicians meet with pharmaceutical representatives four times a month.

Studies also reveal that most physicians erroneously believe the representatives do not influence prescribing habits.

How could anyone NOT be influenced by such a "full-court press"?

As I searched the Internet, hoping to find a few rigorous medical research reports on the use of HBO, I saw a number of references combining "stroke" and "oxygen" in such highly reputable medical journals as *Lancet, Stroke,* and *Journal of Neurology.* Many of the papers described brain and nerve injuries that had been successfully treated, but they had all been discounted, just brushed aside. Why? I wondered. I was dismayed to learn these successful HBO reports have been blatantly ignored as either "too small," or "not yet been replicated enough times" by other scientists. It's true that documentation is essential for any new treatment. Cunningham's refusal to write up his results certainly led to his downfall. There are always "doubting Thomases" who need to see for themselves the results of any new treatment, but according to Dr. Robert Kagan, Medical Director of the MRI Scan Center of Medical Diagnostic Services of America, it is now possible to actually *show* the effect of hyperbaric oxygen on an injured brain *during the treatment.* (Chapter 9 discusses the imaging capabilities of SPECTs, MRIs, and other innovative medical equipment.)

This fact brings forth new questions.

How can anyone deny the "hard" evidence of MRI and SPECT records? Those records clearly demonstrate changes in the brain's metabolic activity. How can any ethical physician continue to demand large, random-controlled, double-blind, placebo-controlled tests for an ailment with as many variables as a stroke?

Every stroke is different, depending on where a clot lodges, or a blood vessel leaks in a tightly packed brain. Each of our ten billion or more neurons has a specific task that only that nerve cell is programmed to perform. With ten billion neurons, and all ten billion of those cells interacting with one another, it's nearly impossible to imagine the quadrillions of possible combinations. Even with someone having a stroke every fifty-three seconds in the United States, it would be hard to assemble enough precisely matched data by race, age, location of infarct and level of health, male or female stroke patients to successfully create a large enough, randomized, cross-over, placebo-controlled stroke study to satisfy every possible "standardized" requirement.

Here's another critical question.

Who would agree to being included in the "placebo" or untreated group when even a few minutes delay means the death of additional brain cells and crippling, life-altering damage. It wouldn't be decent or moral to even ask a patient to make such a sacrifice. Aren't doctors asking too much when they say they want more scientifically rigorous, double-blind tests that would include enormous numbers of precisely matched acute stroke patients?

Both worlds agree: "Stroke Treatment is an Emergency." And a safe, scientifically valid treatment is already available. A treatment with results that have been precisely measured and reported is already available and being used worldwide. Surely, "stroke" is an appropriate medical condition for "anecdotal," off-label, or treatment of choice, for accepting reports of "what has worked" and "how well," with the numbers to back it up, including rigorous follow-up studies. Follow-ups are easy. Hospital records hold the charts of thousands of newly-handicapped stroke survivors who had not been treated within twenty-four hours. Those hundreds of thousands of untreated stroke victims could be matched up with patients who have been treated with either tPA or HBO or both.

Stroke Reports from the Hyperbaric World

Among the HBO physicians who have published their results, I found N. Nighohossian, et al. saying in 1997:

> *Here are the results we've seen in 400 cases*
> Journal of the Neurological Sciences,
> 150(1):27-31, 1997

Four hundred cases, published in 1997! Any physician could be forgiven for saying he hasn't had time to read the report, that this information is "too new" to have become a part of standard accepted practice, but as long ago as 1980 Drs. Neubauer and End reported on:

Hyperbaric oxygen as an adjunct therapy in strokes due to thrombosis, review of 122 patients
Stroke, 11(3): 297–300, May-June 1980

That's one hundred and twenty-two people treated with HBO more than twenty years ago, and Neubauer reported on thirty-two additional stroke patients in 1982 (*Seventh Ann Conf Clin Appl HBO,* Anaheim, California, June 9–11, 1982). He has SPECT scans that show exactly what was happening inside their brains before and after every treatment. He has continued to publish papers describing successfully treating strokes through the 1980s and 1990s. His latest paper, *High dose oxygen therapy in stroke,* was included in the Fifth Congress of the European Federation of Neurological Societies, Copenhagen, Denmark, October 14–18, 2000.

Surely, if a physician claims to be a neurologist, such a physician has had plenty of time to become aware of successfully treated strokes during the past twenty years. It is well known that treating stroke is a matter of preventing or treating brain and nerve damage. Treatments have been reported at conferences and in the professional journals of his claimed area of expertise.

"But Neubauer is only one doctor," you might argue. "Has anyone replicated those results?"

Another physician's report on the Internet:

Nothing can prevent the damage done by the infarct (the original clot) but we have minimized, and sometimes even prevented, any secondary swelling and resultant tissue destruction in the ischemic penumbra when a patient was treated within the first twenty-four hours.

Conventional Medicine

What role is our government playing in health care?

Medicaid paid most of my medical bills, so I wanted to know the government's position on stroke treatment. The National Institutes of Health (NIH) is our government's official organization for investigating and supervising America's health care. I learned that our nation spends a great deal of money on health care. Billions! The National Institute of Health's official report says the federal government paid *$43 billion dollars* on strokes in 2001—that breaks down to $28 billion in cash paid to doctors and hospitals for stroke care and therapy. An additional $15 billion was estimated as lost wages and productivity. Those figures do <u>not</u> include the enormous amount of out-of-pocket money spent on additional Medicare-denied services or treatments, or the extra family expenses. The billion dollars probably does not include the wages lost when a family member has to stop working outside the home so she or he can take care of the stroke victim. It means a family loses two incomes—that of the stroke victim, and that of his or her full-time caretaker.

I found a thorough and thoughtfully written thirty-seven page, single-spaced paper on strokes at the National Institutes of Health website. *Stroke: Hope Through Research* describes the many different kinds of strokes; offers information on recognizing and diagnosing the symptoms of an acute stroke; analyzes the cost of strokes to the government; discusses the risk factors and available treatments, including currently approved medications, surgeries, and rehabilitation therapies; and offers information about special at-risk groups and current clinical trials. I didn't find a single word about oxygen in the available treatments, and none of the current trials included an oxygen component.

There was not even a single mention of a potentially money-saving, brain-saving therapy that might, or could, or should, be investigated in spite of the following statement (page 3):

> *Brain cells die when they no longer receive oxygen and nutrients from the blood...Ischemia is the term used to describe the loss of oxygen and nutrients for brain cells when there is inadequate blood flow...*
>
> *Some brain cells die immediately, while others...make up the ischemic penumbra and can linger in a compromised state for several hours. With timely treatment these cells can be saved...*
>
> National Institutes of Health,
> last reviewed July 1, 2001

The only "hyperbaric oxygen" citation I could locate at that time was in the NIH's multiple sclerosis section. The comment was, "HBO had not successfully cured the disease." I was appalled when I read it. No one has claimed that pressurized oxygen could *cure* this nerve-destructive auto-immune disease. A cure has not yet been found for multiple sclerosis, but there was nothing in the NIH's multiple sclerosis section about

Great Britain's 300-plus HBO clinics *that have provided more than 10,000 treatments to slow down the progress of MS and alleviate the symptoms.*

I have a friend who has just been told that she has MS. When she asked, her doctor said he knew nothing about Great Britain's use of HBO. She is toying with the problems and difficulties that would be involved if she were to move to England—a daunting task for a fragile, elderly widow.

In as much as the NIH is the official government health care branch, what can be done about the lack of HBO use for U.S. citizens?

Politicians who campaign for the right to represent us every election year, the men and women who decide how to spend our tax money for us, repeat as if it were a mantra: *"We have to protect Medicare. We've gotta save Medicare."*

But do they mean it?

Perhaps our elected representatives don't realize that our nation is spending many unnecessary billions of dollars on strokes.

In the chapter discussing the many additional uses of oxygen, it is apparent that we could possibly save so many lives, prevent much unnecessary surgery, heal wounds faster, and save a great deal of money if every regional hospital in America had a hyperbaric facility available for rapidly treating hypoxic emergencies— premature births, automobile crash victims, burns, heart attacks, acute strokes, and for such chronic conditions as burns and hypoxic crush injuries, cerebral palsy, chronic stroke recovery, and slowing the symptoms of multiple sclerosis, in addition to the current fourteen Medicaid-approved uses.

The NIH says they expect to spend at least $28 billion annually on the doctors, therapists, and hospitals needed by stroke victims. Wouldn't it be sensible for this national agency in charge of the nation's health care to at least *investigate* the *published reports* of a safe, non-invasive therapy for brain and nerve damage?

The Public Medical Agencies We Support with Our Donations

The American Heart Association/American Stroke Association (AHA/ASA), in a press release dated February 5, 1998, posted the following statement:

> *There may be a lower cost solution to fighting stroke that doesn't involve new equipment or new therapies...Gaining familiarity with stroke and the treatments available for it—such as the use of clot-busting drugs—may be the best possible result for an acute stroke team.*

Personally, I question why "new equipment" and "new therapies" should be avoided in stroke care. Today large hospitals think it's appropriate to have sensitive, expensive new equipment available, and they hire well-trained personnel to use those instruments. That's what "progress" is all about.

A large hospital recently advertised on TV about the purchase of a new imaging machine, saying, "When we couldn't see it, we couldn't treat it." Well, it has been possible for the last ten or more years for doctors to see what's going on inside a living brain.

Magnetic Resonance Imaging (MRI) equipment is now available in most of the hospitals and trauma centers throughout the nation. Why not use it for stroke patients?

In contrast, compare the criteria outlined for patient inclusion in the DIAS phase II/III nationwide study of acute ischemic stroke, the clinical trial for one of the new clot-busting drugs that has been developed by a hopeful biopharmaceutical firm:

> *The (drug being tested) study in Acute Ischemic Stroke is a global, placebo-controlled, randomized Phase II/III study in acute ischemic stroke. The objective is to assess the efficacy and safety of intravenous use of (the drug) in patients with acute ischemic stroke, administered within 3-9 hours after onset of symptoms.*
>
> *The aim of this diagnostic use of MRI and subsequent patient selection is to detect those patients with the best chances to benefit from thrombolytic therapy.*
>
> *The MRI image has the ability, early after stroke onset, to distinguish normal brain tissue from tissue irreversibly damaged as the result of a stroke. In addition, however, it can identify and quantify the amount of brain tissue which, while not functioning normally, is nevertheless being kept alive by collateral or adjacent blood flow. Only patients with this so-called mismatch (an area of brain which can be salvaged by restoration of blood flow) can be expected to benefit from the intervention.*
>
> *...all follow-up and efficacy endpoints are based on well-accepted clinical scales validated in earlier clinical trials with other stroke therapies.*

You will note that MRIs are required for the study of this experimental new drug. The drug being tested nationwide is a new therapy. Isn't this the very thing the American Stroke Association says is "not needed"?

Furthermore, the American Stroke Association (ASA), a branch of the American Heart Association, claims their mission is "to inform the public." However, a recent survey found that ninety-seven percent of Americans don't know how to recognize the early symptoms of a developing stroke. I was part of that ninety-seven percent. I did realize that I might be having a stroke, but I'd never seen a "public service" announcement describing stroke symptoms on TV nor had I ever heard a public warning on the radio or TV about those short three hours when a stroke can be treated. I'd never even seen a news story describing the symptoms of a stroke, or a billboard message to alert me. Neither had I read an article in any popular magazine explaining what happens during a stroke, or the lasting after-effects of brain damage. Although every one of those agencies said strokes are the third leading cause of death, and the leading cause of crippling disabilities in our nation, there seemed to be a dearth of public knowledge.

The America Heart Association recently announced, "one out of every two American women will die of cardiovascular disease" (a term that includes both heart attacks and strokes). Compare that with the frequently heard "one woman in twenty-seven will die of breast cancer." Have you ever been asked to "walk" or to "run" for stroke? Have you ever received a heart-wrenching letter asking for more stroke research money? Have you ever seen any public warnings about America's leading cause of disability?

The American Stroke Association's website held no information on the subtle ways a stroke can sneak up on you. Nothing about the penumbra and the secondary devastation that can be prevented, but another of their press releases stated that the AHA/ASA:

> *Spends more on stroke-related research and stroke programs than any other non-profit organization... We are second only to the federal government.*

None of the public information says exactly how *much* AHA/ASA is spending on strokes and how much on research. Nor do they publish "who" is giving those huge "private" donations, although the pharmaceutical industry reluctantly acknowledges that they maintain the sixth largest lobbying organization in the nation. They may not like telling you, but AHA/ASA was legally required to reveal the fact that some of their researchers are also "paid consultants" for the pharmaceutical industry.

The only public hint of possible wrongdoing appeared in the required listing of one member of the ASA's Brain Attack Committee, the committee responsible for recommending the standard protocol for stroke treatment throughout the nation, as a "paid consultant" for the firm that manufactures tPA. Several newer, safer, clot-busting drugs with a longer treatment window have been okayed by the FDA, according to reports on the Internet, but tPA is still the *only* recommended, officially approved acute stroke treatment.

If this were the situation in the financial world, where investors deal with something as important as "money," I believe this American Heart Association spokesman, and all other "paid consultants" for pharmaceutical firms, those same health-care professionals who are setting medical standards for this nation, would be questioned about a "conflict of interest," or even a "suppression of trade."

In their *Guidelines for the Management of Patients with Acute Ischemic Stroke,* last updated in 1998, the AMA/ASA Brain Attack Coalition writes:

> *The rules (of evidence) give greater credence to the results of well-designed clinical trials than to anecdotal case reports or case series...*
>
> *The target audience of this statement is primary care physicians, emergency room physicians, and neurologists who care for patients during the first few hours after stroke...also for the education of the general public and for...emergency medical services personnel.*

There you have it.

This respected medical institution was telling all American doctors to follow their protocol, or "Treatment of Choice," and they openly admit to dismissing any and all reports of strokes *successfully* treated with HBO. Just brushing these Unprofitable Modalities (UMs) aside, calling them "merely anecdotal."

And I found this bit of advice in the AHA/ASA's *Emergent Supportive Care and Treatment of Acute Complications* section:

> *Maintaining adequate tissue oxygenation is an important component of emergent management. Hypoxia results in anaerobic metabolism and depletion of energy stores that can increase the extent of brain injury and worsen outcome...<u>No data establish the benefit of supplemental oxygen, and there is no reason to routinely administer this therapy</u>... Hyperbaric oxygen may be useful for the occasional patient with stroke (that is) secondary to air embolism, <u>but its role in the general treatment of acute ischemic stroke has not been adequately tested.</u>*

When I read that, my blood pressure almost exploded!

Your money and mine, our donations, support the American Heart Association/American Stroke Association. The AHA spokesmen agree that the brain's need for additional oxygen during a stroke has been clearly demonstrated and yet they officially discourage emergency room doctors from even giving their patients everyday, unpressurized, available medical oxygen that could protect endangered, but still undamaged, brain tissues.

As an untreated, disabled stroke-survivor, I find that statement, and the official attitude of the American Heart/American Stroke Association to be dishonest, arrogant, and offensive. I speak from my own experience when I tell you that living with the after-effects of an untreated minor stroke is very unpleasant. Drugs like tPA may eventually be one answer, but they will never be the only answer to the crippling effects of oxygen deprivation.

On the Internet, I found these chilling paralysis figures and numbers:

Hemiparesis (weakness on one side of the body) limits 227,000 people and is of low primacy. Similarly in hemiplegia (paralysis on one side of the body) 79 percent of cases are caused by stroke and 10 percent by injury. Partial paralysis in an upper extremity limits activity for 80,000 people. Stroke is the cause for 71 percent of cases. Paraparesis (partial paralysis, usually affecting only the legs), limits activity for 51,000 people, of which 61 percent are caused by stroke. Other types of partial paralysis of a lower extremity limit activity for 73,000 people, most of whom are paralyzed in one leg (65,000). The rest in one foot or both feet...with 60 percent of cases caused by stroke. Paralysis in other sites, complete or partial, limits 180,000.

Altogether, paralysis (loss of voluntary movement) limits 1.1 million people, usually the result of stroke.

More than a million damaged moms, dads, babies, grandmas, and grandpas—that really puts a face on the figures. Arms and legs that will no longer move—and most of those frustrating disabilities caused by strokes, or "breaks" in the connection between mind and muscle.

How can the American Heart Association tell a million crippled people "don't be depressed," when so many of our kindly, caring doctors still refuse to even consider using a well-documented, safe, non-invasive, and frequently successful stroke treatment? How can our generously supported public institutions, organizations that we trust because they are the "experts," ignore a treatment as basic as delivering oxygen to the brain, when the entire medical world agrees that it is the ischemic penumbra, that "vicious cycle of swelling," that's *responsible for causing seventy to eighty-five percent of stroke disability?*

7

WHAT I GLEANED FROM THE NET

I wanted to know exactly what "stroke" meant in the medical world, so I turned to a medical dictionary:

An area of moderately ischemic brain tissue surrounding an area of more severe ischemia; blood flow to this area may be enhanced in order to prevent the spread of cerebral infarction.

Dorland's Illustrated Medical Dictionary, 28th ed., 1994

I found a description of a thrombolitic (clot) stroke on a chat-line and after reading it, I could understand why my urine had smelled so vile for a day or two, why I'd been so thirsty and had to use the restroom so often. My kidneys must have been valiantly trying to clear my blood of a sludge of dead cells and devastating biochemicals.

In 1998 Peter Allen had written:

The five chemical steps in any stroke have been the subject of intensive research. Briefly, they are:
Step 1. the oxygen and glucose supply falls.
Step 2. cells generate acids such as lactic acid, which in turn leads to cellular swelling and a disturbance in the movement of ions such as

sodium and potassium. The cell then depolarizes (loses the electrical charge in their membranes).

Step 3. As a result of depolarization, calcium floods the area, causing the release of excessive amounts of the neurotransmitter glutamate, which binds to the glutamate receptors on neighboring cells.

Step 4. The excess glutamate leads to over-excitation in the nerve cells and further rounds of ion movement and functional loss.

During the three hour window of opportunity while this is taking place, restoring blood flow with tPA is one way to save cells, but another way is to interrupt the above process with so-called "neuroprotective" drugs. There are drugs in the pipeline, (my informant says) that will stabilize the cell membrane, reduce their excitability, mop up damaging chemicals, or have anti-inflammatory actions. There are about seven drugs in various stages of development, and another three that have been dropped as their results were not entirely satisfactory.

Step 5. Now the internal structures of a cell begin to fail, fatty acids are converted into inflammatory molecules, and highly reactive free radicals are formed —all of which cumulates in the death of the nerve cell. In effect, the injured cells self-destruct.

Although there have been some early disappointments with neuroprotecting drugs, there remains great conviction as to their value, and researchers believe there are sound reasons to hope they can and will work. It is expected that this area will remain one of great research and clinical activity for the foreseeable future.

"There are drugs in the pipeline," Allen had written in 1998. By the time I read his description, it was 2001, so I revisited the American Heart/Stroke website looking for the names of those new drugs that were going to control stroke damage. The only treatment the American Stroke Association was recommending was still the Genentech-manufactured tPA, the three-hour time-limited, clot-dissolving thrombolitic enzyme. Here was the ASA's suggested 2001 protocol (according to their statement, "The largest audience for this paper includes neurologists, emergency physicians, primary care physicians, neurosurgeons and vascular surgeons who care for persons seen within the first few hours"):

THROMBOLYTIC THERAPY: Measures to expedite clot lysis (dissolve it) and restore circulation which may limit the extent of brain injury and improve outcome after stroke...

Available thrombolitic drugs include recombinant tissue plasminogen activator (rtPA), streptokinase, p-anisoylated lys-plasminogen-streptokinase activator complex, urokinase and p-anisoylated lys-plasminogen-streptokinase activator complex, urokinase, and prourokinase. Supplemental techniques include mechanical clot disruption, pulse spray delivery, distal clot delivery, modifications in catheter design, and administration of heparin or lys-plasminogen may improve the likelihood of

recanalization (rebuilding of damaged capillaries).
No technique has been shown to be better than others.

By 2003, I found much more information—a comprehensive list of stroke articles on the AHA site, including one on the experimental use of hyperbaric oxygen on rats, but not a word about Dr. Neubauer, or other physicians who had successfully treated patients.

Neuroprotectants?

I'd found a number of reports on the use of the blood thinners, aspirin and Warfarin, and many reports on the pros and cons of tPA in the usual discussions of stroke drug approvals, but nothing on neuroprotectants until I read a report on a substance being tested for slowing down the progression of Parkinson's. I was curious. I know Parkinson's is a disease involving nerve damage, so I looked it up and found that John Ely, Ph.D., Research Professor of Radiation Studies, emeritus, at the University of Washington, had a lot to say about strokes and neuroprotectants.

In the *Journal of Orthomolecular Medicine* 13(2):105–9, 1998, Dr. Ely had written:

> *...In 29 years of animal stroke studies, one substance that afforded a markedly higher degree of protection than all others tested was a normal endogenous molecule, CoEnzyme Q10. Because of increasing worldwide use of Q10 we were able serendipitously to report on possibly the first observation of a human recovering almost completely from an unexpected cerebral hemorrhage following*

four weeks of pretreatment with Q10 at a pharmacological dose commonly employed for a wide variety of disorders. Clearly, clinical studies are needed to confirm the significance of our observed result...The safety and efficiency of CoQ10 has already been proven in nine large scale international trials in cardiomyopathy, etc., and its apparent benefits in numerous disorders, including AIDS and possibly aging itself. However, the confirmation should be done in trials specifically designed for stroke...If confirmed, this result does not diminish the urgent need for development of synthetic stroke agents, but may facilitate their realization by decreasing the protective functions needed from the agents.

Ely has been studying the action of CoEnzyme Q10 since 1971 and writes:

In three animal models (dog, rat, gerbil) ubiquinone (CoEnzyme Q10) was the only agent giving complete protection and this was over two times more often than the next best agent (naloxone) of the many tested to date. Some of the animals were pretreated and some post-stroke (less than 12 hours).

He explains that in 2000 he had attended the annual winter meeting of the American Stroke Association and witnessed the reported failures of three new drugs that had been in human stage testing by large pharmaceutical companies attempting to create commercial, patentable brain-protectants. Such failures had cost the firms enormous amounts of time and money. Ely adds that he has seen at least fifty such neuroprotectants that have failed during the last decade, and suggests that physicians administer CoEnzyme Q10 to prevent or at least to limit stroke damage until the drug companies do succeed in producing a more effective synthetic neuroprotectant. He ends an urgent message in the June 2000 issue of *Orthomolecular Medicine* by writing:

> *We emphasize that we are not advising people to self-treat. However, everyone must realize that each year in the U.S. alone, over 650,000 families have a loved one hospitalized for stroke...The families have a right to know that CoEnzyme Q10 exists in their health food stores.*

Dr. Ely asks any physician who uses CoQ10 to treat a stroke patient to "report by e-mail *(apresi@aol.com)*, giving the patient's identification, date of stroke, treating stroke center, prognosis, time delay before ubiquinone (swallowed or intubation), dosage including other agents, and progress up to 4 weeks post-stroke."

Another common, readily available neuroprotectant was reported in September, 2003, on *WebMDhealth.* Catherine Neto, Ph.D., of the University of Massachusetts, reported at the American Chemical Society's meeting in Washington, DC, that cranberry extract was found to reduce brain cell damage by 50 percent when given to laboratory rats immediately after a stroke. She says further tests are required before the researchers will be able to suggest the proper dosage for humans. In the meantime, the National Institutes of Health advises, "lower your blood pressure, stop smoking, and control diabetes and heart disease." Not very helpful advice for someone who is having a stroke, but it is worth knowing that if all else fails you can ask a family member or friend to bring you some CoQ10 and/or cranberry juice while you are in the hospital and your stroke is stabilizing.

Surgeries

Maybe you would rather try surgery to prevent a second stroke? The AMA suggests that if you've already had a stroke within the past one hundred and twenty days, and one of your neck's carotid arteries is found to be clogged from seventy to ninety-five percent, your physician might suggest a "carotid endartectomy." In such an operation the surgeon would delicately scrape out the waxy material (cholesterol) that is clogging the carotid artery. This operation would reduce chances of a second stroke from one in four to less than one in ten, according to reports in *Stroke* (June 1991) and the *New England Journal of Medicine* (Aug. 1991). Follow-up of twenty-four patients found that only five percent of the surgically treated patients died during the following eighteen months, while twelve percent of the patients died who had been treated only with medicine.

As I read these stories, I couldn't help wondering why a study of twenty-four surgical patients was considered significant while the reports from Dr. Neubauer and other physicians who have treated more than a thousand acute strokes with hyperbaric oxygen have been ignored.

Dr. Neubauer included in his study a description of the stickiness, or adhesiveness, of red or white blood cells and the way they stick to platelets in the endothelium (the membrane lining blood vessels). The AHA/ASA 2001 protocol said nothing about prescribing aspirin or other blood thinners to reduce the "stickiness" of blood cells, although aspirin therapy is recommended as standard treatment in Great Britain. When I visited the ASA website in 2002, I noted that Bayer Aspirin had sponsored their 2000 Stroke Challenge program, so I assume aspirin is now included in the AMA/ASA's latest emergency protocols.

I did not find the word "oxygen" anywhere in their 2002 "acute stroke" protocol, although they were writing about brain cells that die without oxygen. The *only* treatment this group was advising physicians to use when treating an acute stroke was still tPA.

A recent (*JAMA*, 8/22/01) report from the University of California at San Francisco warned that too-high levels of *homocysteine,* a protein normally present in blood, can thicken and cause clots which, in turn, can lead to heart attacks and strokes. I found no suggestion that testing stroke-prone patients for raised homocysteine levels might be valuable; not a single word about homocysteine in the public advice given by AHA/ASA. I would think an assessment of a known risk-factor would be helpful for any doctor. As for me, I remember reading that vitamin B controls the production of homocysteine. I now include a vitamin B complex tablet along with my CoQ10 capsule in my daily batch of vitamins as a simple precaution.

Some Current Stroke Treatments

The National Institute of Neurological Disorders and Stroke, a division of the AMA/ASA, reports: "rtPA has been successfully used in Europe, Australia and Italy on 333 patients treated within three hours of onset"; the report concludes:

> *Despite hemorrhages, the rate of death or severe disability was less in the actively treated group...only six percent of all stroke patients receive tPA.*

Six percent? Is that what they call "success"? What do they call the ninety-four percent who either died or were severely disabled?

Here's what I call success:

> *My son Michael had a stroke last year at the age of 5. The stroke took half his brain. Due to prayer and HBOT he now has the ability to move his arm, some use of his fingers and almost complete speech back after 87 HBOT treatments. They did so much for him. This was a child who was not supposed to ever again breathe, talk, walk or eat. Much less live.*
>
> From: hbo-list@lists.best.com, Aug 7, 2000

This internet report is also a tribute to a child's body's ability to heal itself when given a little help.

Dr. Neubauer is sometimes referred to as "an American pioneer in the use of hyperbaric oxygen for treating an acute stroke." He says his current acute stroke protocol follows medically established scientific double-blind standards. Neubauer's patients have

111

Some received only tPA, some were treated only with hyperbaric oxygen and a third group received both. Every patient was given a SPECT scan before and after each treatment to measure metabolic activity in the brain. Those who were given HBO were treated for one hour at 1.5 ATA every six hours around the clock until the stroke had stabilized, receiving a total of ten to twenty HBO treatments. The mortality rate was about the same for each group. Stroke is, after all, the third leading cause of death, but Neubauer's report found the disabilities and long-term care were significantly lower for his HBO patients.

This is what I call success:

Neubauer tells the story of a seventy-seven-year-old man who had just been diagnosed as having a stroke. The man arrived at the clinic with increasing right-side weakness, dizziness, confusion, and swallowing difficulties (symptoms of an average-intensity thrombolitic stroke). HBO was administered within two hours of his arrival. He was treated as an outpatient, receiving two hyperbaric oxygen treatments a day for a total of sixteen treatments. At that time his SPECT scan showed only minimal neurological deficits. Three months later he was given a follow-up SPECT scan that showed a normal brain pattern! He had no crippling disabilities!

In *Hyperbaric Medicine Today*, Feb, 2001, Dr. Neubauer called hyperbaric oxygen the treatment of choice for acute strokes because of the rapid physiological effects of hyperbaric oxygen. His article concludes by listing the following advantages of giving oxygen within a four-hour time frame:

1) It reduces cerebral edema—focal and generalized.
2) It overcomes ischemic hypoxia, thus stopping or reducing the ischemic cascade.
3) It protects the integrity of the cell membrane and restores the integrity of the blood-brain barrier.
4) It neutralizes toxic amines.
5) It neutralizes free radicals.
6) It reduces the adhesiveness of the red cell and stickiness of the platelets in the endothelium.
7) It efficiently elevates the driving force (plasma flow) for oxygen, making increasing tissue space availability.
8) It reactivates dormant, idling hypoxic neurons.
9) It reduces lactate peaks.

I wish I'd been living in south Florida when I had my "minor" stroke, and that I'd been so stroke-savvy that I'd have gone immediately to Dr. Neubauer's Ocean Hyperbaric Center at Lauderdale-by-the-Sea for treatment. Or that my own local hospital had known and followed his effective protocol, but I live on the other side of the continent, in a state that doesn't list even one hyperbaric oxygen facility and doesn't believe we need one. As our local neurologist recently told one of my friends, "I haven't seen any good science to validate the 'oxygen' theory."

This was from a man who considers himself as a "nerve specialist."

As long ago as 1980, Neubauer reported in *Stroke*, 11(3):297–300, a highly-respected medical journal, on his successful use of hyperbaric oxygenation on 122 patients. Today his Ocean Hyperbaric Center continues to treat stroke patients. He speaks frequently at international symposiums to tell other physicians about the strokes he has treated successfully at his clinic. I can't help comparing Neubauer's intelligent use of new medical technology with our local "specialist," and being reminded of the old folk-saying, "there are none so blind as those who will not see."

Neubauer is not alone in his belief in oxygenation.

Dr. Steenblock, Director of the Health Restoration Center in Mission Viejo, California, at his Health Restoration website, gets very technical in his discussion of a stroke's biochemical aspects:

> *Repeat multitracer PET (positron emission tomography) studies with human stroke victims have shown viable tissue in the border zone of ischemia for up to 48 hours after the cerebrovascular attack. Interventions to improve ischemic resistance should aim at improving the oxygen supply.*
>
> *Red blood cell clumping, platelet aggregation, endothelial swelling, increased blood and plasma viscosity are just some of the factors that contribute to the decrease in the flow of red cells through ischemic tissue capillaries.*
>
> *Plasma, on the other hand, has been shown to reach all ischemic and post-ischemic capillaries and is able to pass through capillaries where red blood cells can no longer move, due to the restrictive changes created by the ischemic process...It is possible to dissolve sufficient oxygen in plasma to meet the needs of the brain.*

114

Thus, in the acute stroke patient, the use of hyperbaric oxygen can provide oxygen to ischemic neurons and keep them alive while fibrinolytic mechanisms (tPA) are brought to bear on the cerebral thrombosis causing the ischemia. This results in the salvage of the ischemic penumbra to a degree impossible with any other therapy.

After carefully studying and analyzing all of this information, I'm angry about the way my medical team treated my stroke.

I think you would be angry, too, if you were one of those 700,000 Americans who will have a crippling stroke this year (that's more than one every minute of the day), and neither you nor your doctor has ever heard of hyperbaric oxygen or CoQ10.

Unless, of course, you recognized the earliest symptoms of a stroke and were close enough to a knowledgeable Stroke Center to arrive in time for the experts to run a series of tests and administer tPA, the clot-dissolving enzyme, within the first three hours of your attack.

Oxygen is so basic, so safe. And seems so obvious.

A brilliant physicist like Professor Teller can't be wrong when he says, "This is 'good science'." Personally, I don't believe Dr. Neubauer is spreading false hope when he says we should quickly "give the brain oxygen."

Cold Therapy—An "Off Label" or "Compassionate Use" Treatment

During the last few years hypothermia, or "cold therapy," triggered by animal experiments and the experiences of people who have either fallen into icy waters or been injured while out in frigid weather, has emerged. Doctors have noticed that when people are chilled, the body's metabolism is slowed, the brain's use of oxygen is temporarily reduced, and this slows the production of nerve-killing chemicals and stabilizes the nearby cell membranes.

A neurologist at Duke University's Intensive Care Unit of the Stroke and Trauma Center, hoping to effectively treat an acute stroke, reasoned that "swelling is swelling." Just as ice-packs are useful for reducing and limiting swelling, as every coach, nurse, and doctor knows, if dying brain cells create additional swelling in the brain, why not, he thought, try hypothermia—chilling a stroke patient during the first twenty-four hours, before the brain *really* starts to swell, before secondary swelling creates such severe pressure inside the skull that fragile brain tissues are squeezed into the brain stem, destroying the control center of the body—the site of consciousness, breathing, and heartbeat.

One such "compassionate use" or "off-label" experiment was reported by Jon Franklin, science reporter for the *News and Observer* of Raleigh, North Carolina, in 2001.

For three days the patient, who had been admitted while having a moderate stroke caused by a clot in her left middle cerebral artery, was chilled to 91.5 degrees Fahrenheit. After eight weeks in and out of the hospital's neurointensive care unit and several life-threatening bouts with pneumonia, after having been cared for by a multitude of nurses, technicians, respiratory therapists, pharmacologists, neurologists, and a constant parade of experts at a cost of hundreds of thousands of dollars, she was discharged from the hospital two months later. She spent another two months in a rehabilitation center learning to stand without assistance, to walk again, to feed herself, and to go to the bathroom before she could go home, and continue an intense program of physical therapy for the next two years. She is grateful to be alive after such an ordeal; she can manage her home once again, but many of her abilities are gone forever.

Wouldn't it have been simpler, more effective, less costly and life-threatening if that vast army of medical experts had either been aware of and had access to oxygen's healing qualities, as reported by Dr. Neubauer, or had even known that oxygen, when delivered under pressure can:

Reduce cerebral edema (brain swelling)

Reduce intracranial pressure

Elevate oxygen's diffusional driving force, thus increasing oxygen availability

Restore the integrity of the blood-brain barrier and cell membranes

Dissolve oxygen in cerebrospinal fluid

Neutralize toxic cellular byproducts

Scavenge free radicals

Promote function of immune cells

This "experiment" was at Duke University, which has had an active hyperbaric oxygen program since 1963, with more than a thousand published research papers.

Among my collection of reports and studies are several current press announcements from four medical industry firms announcing their new or ongoing tests for ingenious new methods for cooling a patient down.

What I'm waiting to read is a newspaper story hailing HBO as a major stroke "breakthrough," administered as an "off label" or "compassionate care" treatment for an acute thrombolitic stroke in a major hospital.

Dracula to the Rescue?

In early 2003, a story was widely reported that a "new and better" drug for acute stroke treatment had just been identified. The substance that is released when a vampire bat bites a victim contains a powerful clot-dissolving protein known as *Desmondus rotundus* salivary plasminogen activator, or DSPA. It is a clot dissolver that is declared to be hundreds of times faster and much safer than tPA, but some members of the medical world seem to be having a difficult time accepting a replacement for tPA.

The results of tests on mice, using a new synthetic version of bat saliva, were announced by Australian researcher Dr. Robert Medcalf of Monash University, Victoria, Australia, on January 10, 2003. Medcalf suggested that DSPA can safely be given as long as *nine* hours after a stroke. It did not harm two brain receptor cells that have sometimes been damaged by tPA, although reports of tPA damage still continue to be controversial.

Dr. Wolf-Dieter Schieuning of the PAION GmbH biopharmaceutical firm of Aachen, Germany, the firm that researched bat saliva and produced this synthetic version, told reporters the company chose the anticoagulant found in vampire bat saliva, rather than that of leeches or ticks, because bat saliva more precisely targets blood clots by specifically dissolving fibrinogen, the mesh-like structure that holds a blood clot together. DSPA is currently in phase II/III human trials in Europe and Asia and in ten or more hospitals in the United States. Dr. Anthony Furlan of the Cleveland Clinic Foundation of Cleveland, Ohio, director of the American trials, calls DSPA "the most effective clot buster we've ever seen. When given within the first nine hours, it can reverse paralysis, reverse blindness, restore a patient's ability to speak, and restore a stroke victim to a relatively normal lifestyle."

But despite such glowing reports, an eminent neurologist on the staff of New York University School of Medicine told a *New York Times* reporter who asked for his opinion, "The nine-hour window is not necessarily an advantage... Any drug administered after three hours is essentially pointless because the damage has already been done."

It would appear this eminent professor is not aware of the measured, progressive, secondary damage that is unnecessarily inflicted on a victim during a stroke.

Bayer Biological Products and the University of California at Los Angeles reported in 9/2001 in the *Journal of Thrombosis & Haemostasis* on the effectiveness of plasmin, a natural protein derived from human plasma, as a clot-buster. The researchers reported that plasmin was just as effective as tPA in rapidly dissolving blood clots in rabbits, and much safer. In a completely blocked blood vessel, plasmin dissolved more of the blood clot and restored blood flow, while an equivalent dose of tPA dissolved less of the clot and did not restore blood flow. When administered in partially blocked vessels, plasmin and tPA dissolved the existing blockage equally well. Using ear puncture rebleed on further studies, the researchers measured the effects of plasmin and tPA on rebleeding. Equal doses of either plasmin or tPA were administered over fifty-five minutes by catheter. Nine out of ten rabbits receiving tPA showed fibrinolytic rebleeding. No rabbits receiving plasmin had fibrinogen rebleeding, and the report concluded that plasmin was just as effective and much safer than tPA, and had potential usefulness for humans.

The elapsed time (the old three-hour time frame) between clot formation and administration of either plasmin or tPA was not reported. As of this writing, there have been no further press releases reporting the firm's ability and desire to begin human trials.

New Surgeries and Drugs

Currently on the surgical horizon are a number of new procedures to get oxygen to the brain quickly. Some are shunts (tiny tubes to carry blood and oxygen) through veins and arteries. One such shunt currently in Phase III trials is so tiny that it can be threaded into the smallest of capillaries. Another research hospital has announced a new system for "propping open" arteries. One can only hope that our surgeons and health care system are ready for these challenges.

The Oregonian newspaper, in a story by Oz Hopkins Koglin describing a report given in 2001 to the American Society of Radioneurology in Bu.. Oregon Health Services University researche. described clinical trials using a catheter inserted into a patient's groin and run up to the brain to deliver ultrasound and tPA. This procedure is intended to more efficiently break large clots into smaller pieces, allowing tPA administered at the same time to dissolve the smaller segments. The addition of ultrasound allowed the time of treatment for patients with blockages in the front of the brain to be extended to six hours, and for those occurring in the back of the brain to twenty-four hours. According to the article, after three months half of the patients had recovered sufficiently to resume normal or near-normal activities.

Hope for Hyperbaric Oxygen?

There may be a change in the political future of hyperbaric oxygen. In the spring of 2001, the Texas legislature agreed that brain injuries can be successfully treated with oxygen. The parents of children afflicted with cerebral palsy joined forces with the caretakers of stroke victims to contact lawmakers. Texas lawmakers say they can't remember any measure, ever, that attracted such an enormous volume of citizen support. Along with phone calls and letters, the wife of one stroke survivor used the Internet to urge parents, relatives, and friends to write, call, and/or otherwise send their very active support to the legislators. One representative's startled comment was, "I've never seen such an active response to a measure." The bill says hyperbaric oxygen treatments are approved. In fact, health care insurance providers are mandated to provide HBO on request for oxygen-deprived brains. If Texas can do it, can the rest of the America be far behind?

This is just one example of the way information shared on the Internet and through organized efforts is changing medical practice. Today a patient may actually know more about his or her disease, disability, and potential treatment than anyone but the most research oriented physician. I'm just one example of someone with a disability who searches the Internet, reading and learning everything available about my special problem. I have the time and the desire to learn about every new experiment, to read every report on new research. This is virtually impossible for even the most dedicated physician who is busy with patients, running an office, and trying to have a life in a field that's a bubbling ferment of new directions, new and ever more sophisticated (and expensive) drugs, new equipment, new trials, and new medical approaches to the things that go wrong with our ever-changing bodies.

These are just a few articles among the recent stroke pharmaceutical reports that have come across my computer. I also read all press releases announcing new neuroprotectives, oxygen carriers, hyperthermia, and gene therapies.

Carrying on my personal research on HBO and strokes, I wondered whether Dr. Neubauer and prominent Scottish hyperbaric physician Dr. Philip James agreed with neurosurgeon Dr. K.K. Jain on how to treat an acute stroke.

Yes. Both men say they've stretched that impossibly brief three-hour tPA window. Both agreed that oxygen given later is not nearly so effective in preventing brain damage as oxygen administered during the earliest stages of an active stroke, but both suggested either surgery or drugs in addition to HBO. Both agreed with the advice another American doctor gave on the hyperbaric oxygen web site. "If you have a stroke, it's best to have it only in a clinic or hospital." That made me laugh!

Of course they were right. Most professionals do understand that stroke is a medical emergency; that a rapidly treated patient with immediate access to the best available medicine in a well-run Stroke Center **can** recover completely, as former President Ford did. So did the Broadway singer and dancer Ben Vareen, who has recently been advertising aspirin on television. He says he has completely recovered from a stroke and "it's great to be back." Complete recoveries ARE possible. But how many of us are going to just "happen" to be sitting in a modern, well-equipped hospital with a brain surgeon handy? How many people have access to HBO? How many of us even know that immediately taking an aspirin if you suspect you *might* be having a stroke is a medically approved emergency treatment?

If your physician does suggest surgery, some physicians have used HBO as an adjunct to a carotid endartectomy. A report in *Surgical Neurology* (15(1):43–46, 1981) reported on twenty-two patients given HBO during stroke. Ten of the patients showed improved motor function. Seven were successfully revascularized and had no recurrence of the neurological defects. Three of the patients were not successfully revascularized, and their neurological damage returned. Twelve patients did not respond to

HBO. As with any medical procedure or medicine, no intervention works ALL the time.

Neubauer says the Russians published an acute stroke treatment paper as long ago as 1980, reporting that they had treated more than a thousand "active" strokes within a critical four-hour time period, and detailed the protocol they followed.

Many papers cited in Scandinavian and German literature suggest that the earlier oxygen is administered to a hypoxic brain, the more successfully blood vessels are prevented from swelling.

Dr. R. Veltkamp, in a letter to the *Journal of Neurologic Science* (150, pp 1–2, 1997), goes so far as to advise the emergency use of oxygen in the ambulance, suggesting:

> *...that portable HBO_2 equipment be designed for the initiation of therapy on site by trained personnel before and during <u>emergency transportation to the hospital</u>. The effectiveness of HBO_2 in combination with other new hyperacute stroke therapies can and must be (re)explored.*

A local man suspected he might be having a stroke and when he called 9-1-1, his speech was slurred, he staggered, and his thoughts seemed unfocused. The paramedics gave him oxygen while he was in the ambulance, and his speech difficulties immediately cleared up. Later, in the hospital, while four doctors were working over him, his wife asked why they weren't giving him oxygen, but the four medical "experts" ignored her. Nevertheless, I saw him at a recent function and he'd recovered to the point where he was both speaking and walking easily. Oxygen had protected his brain during the first hour of his attack.

A posting dated Nov. 2000 on *www. Hyperbaricservices.com* sums up everything we've been talking about:

> *HBO_2 helps reduce cerebral edema, which reduces intercranial pressure, improving capillary blood flow, increasing oxygen delivery to tissues with disrupted circulation. HBO_2 helps prevent secondary hypoxic damage.*
>
> *When there is damage to the brain, the trauma, lack of oxygen, and the body's natural inflammatory response leads to the formation of edema. The edema, in turn, leads to further hypoxia that in turn exacerbates the hypoxia...By improving oxygen delivery to the injured and surrounding tissues, and by helping to reduce edema, HBO_2 can interrupt this vicious cycle of hypoxia and edema initiated by the original trauma damage.*

My stroke was called "only minor," but it's hard for me to walk, and my speech is no longer crisp. Is it surprising that I'm envious? Our local doctors may not believe in the "oxygen" theory, but the ambulance paramedics *DO* understand oxygen's healing powers —just everyday hospital oxygen administered under normal pressure. This is a good and sensible reason why I should have called an ambulance when my husband and I suspected that I might be having a stroke.

Unfortunately, it seems that such information is routinely ignored by many of America's leading medical institutions. Maybe the procedure actually relieves the patient's symptoms, but the results are still being scornfully dismissed by many physicians.

There may be hope for our grandchildren, however.

In February of 1997, a group of American doctors, including neurologists and hyperbaric and emergency physicians, met to organize the first phase of a new stroke/HBO study designed to meet every exacting National Institute of Health standard. This project is described in the February, 2001, issue of *Hyperbaric Medicine Today*; it will be under the direction of Dr. Paul Harch of New Orleans, Dr. Toole and Dr. George Howard of the University of Alabama.

This study to examine the effectiveness of hyperbaric oxygen in treating hypoxic brain tissue wasn't organized until 1997. That means, at 750,000 strokes a year, we will see an additional 750,000 crippling strokes times "x" number of years before these rigorously scientific test results can be completed and publicized. Medical researchers work at a deliberate pace; it takes time to organize a rock-solid study. The researchers must accumulate enough victims to match the demographics (age, education, financial status) and risk factors (severity of stroke). These stroke patients will be divided, as Dr. Neubauer's were twenty years ago, into three groups: (1) those who are given oxygen alone, (2) patients given oxygen plus tPA, and (3) those receiving only tPA. The results will be reported and tests replicated by other researchers, their results confirmed by fellow scientists, and the evidence peer reviewed before the results will be published.

In a previous section I wrote about Peter Allen's optimism over neuroprotectant drugs that were "in the pipeline" and his belief that the drug companies were "on the verge" of succeeding. Allen's optimistic report was written more than eight years ago, but I haven't seen any stories in the press or on TV about vitamin B and homocysteine, vampire bat saliva, CoQl0, or cranberries. Admittedly, the cranberries had been tested only on rats, but the CoQ10 proved to be an extremely efficient neuroprotectant in laboratory animals.

Nor have our doctors been told by America's leading medical authorities to *GIVE OXYGEN* to a patient having a stroke. In fact, the authorities have advised *AGAINST* it, although this advice could be changing.

In the American Stroke Association's May/June 2004 issue of *Stroke Connection,* a journal filled with upbeat stories of heroic stroke survivors who rise above their stroke-created disabilities, including such tales as that of one woman who actually completed a 24-mile marathon walk/run, the journal included this interesting piece of stroke information:

> *In a randomized study of eight patients receiving 100 percent oxygen by face mask for eight hours, and four patients who got only room air, when the oxygen was administered within 12 hours of stroke the volume of brain tissue affected by the stroke decreased to 78 percent at three hours, then increased to 114*

percent at 24 hours and 194 percent at one week. In those who got only room air the volume of affected brain tissue increased to 145 percent at three hours, 229 percent at 24 hours and 253 percent at one week. The article concludes that "early hyperoxygen" therapy appears safe and could possibly extend the "time window" for effective therapy after ischemic stroke.

This is a reluctant admission that oxygen, even at normal room pressure, is safe and saves brain cells.

At the current rate of 700,000 strokes per year, with 500,000 of them being first time incidents, unless things change, we will see another three million, five hundred thousand new stroke victims in the next six years.

Why are our doctors still being officially advised to ignore oxygen? What could be more natural, safer, cheaper, and more readily available than oxygen? As an ancient *curandero* in Belize told medical anthropologists, "God gave us a remedy for every disease in the world, if we're only smart enough to use it."

I believe we should *USE* this natural remedy. We really don't need, and don't want, another million or more newly disabled stroke victims.

FINALLY—I GET THE "REAL" SKINNY ON ACUTE STROKES

8

A friend, knowing my interest, gave me a printout of Chapter 17, covering "strokes," from K.K. Jain's *Textbook of Hyperbaric Medicine, 3rd Edition,* a standard reference for HBO providers. At last I had a dependable medical reference I could consult, written by a *bona fide* specialist, a neurosurgeon. Not only did Jain write "the" textbook on hyperbaric medicine, but he is a respected physician/surgeon/researcher who has taught at Harvard, UCLA, and Toronto.

Jain is a firm believer in the use of pressurized oxygen, or HBO, and he explains the science. Oxygen under pressure, he writes, can reduce swelling in the brain, restore a damaged blood-brain vessel's barrier, and stimulate the growth of new blood vessels, as well as clearing free radicals from the bloodstream and reducing the stickiness of white blood cells and platelets.

Dr. Jain writes, "when a patient has a hemorrhagic stroke, the vast majority of doctors and nurses will 'just write the patient off—never will be anything but a vegetable.'"

As you read in the letter in Chapter Four, the quality of life for even a severe hemorrhagic stroke victim can be improved. Her husband matched Jain's dismal profile—a severe "bleed"—and her husband's doctors actively tried to persuade her to "just put him in a nursing home." But when Allene and her husband were married, she did not promise to "love him until he has a stroke." She'd said, "for so long as we both shall live," and thanks to her heroic efforts to get hyperbaric oxygen treatments for this man, she has changed medical practice throughout the entire state of Texas.

Dr. Jain defines "stroke" as:

> *The term normally used to describe the sudden onset of a neurological deficit such as weakness or paralysis due to disturbance of the blood flow to the brain...is loosely used to cover ischemic and hemorrhagic episodes...An ischemic stroke occurs when a thrombus or an embolus blocks an artery to the brain, blocking or reducing the blood flow to the brain, and consequently the transport of oxygen and glucose which are critical elements for brain function.*

Listing the risk factors for "stroke," Jain says, "A major cause is atherosclerosis, a non-inflammatory degenerative disease that can affect almost any artery in the body." After I'd read his complete risk factor list, I realized that just "being alive" can be dangerous to a person's health. Nobody is safe.

He lists the following risk factors:

1. Aging
2. Alcohol
3. Atherosclerosis involving major vessels
   a. Atherosclerosis of aortic arch

  b. Atrial fibrillation
  c. Endocarditis
  d. Left ventricular hypertrophy
  e. Mitral valve prolapse
  f. Myocardial infarction
  g. Patent foramen ovale
4. Coagulation disorders
5. Cold
6. Endocrine disorders
  a. Diabetes Mellitus
  b. Hypothyroidism
7. Genetic
  a. Angiotensin-converting enzyme gene deletion polymorphism
  b. Genetically determined cardiovascular, hematological, and metabolic disorders causing stroke
8. Hemorrheological disturbances
  a. Elevated hematocrit
  b. Increased blood viscosity
  c. Red blood cell disorders
  d. Leukocytosis
9. Heredity: parental history of stroke is associated with stroke risk in the offspring
10. Hyperlipemia
11. Hypertension
12. Hypotension
13. Lack of physical activity
14. Metabolic disorders
  a. Hyperuricemia
  b. Hyperhomocysteinemia
15. Migraine

16. Nutritional disorders
    a. High salt intake
    b. Malnutrition
    c. Vitamin deficiency
17. Obesity
18. Psycho-social factors: anger, aggression, stress
19. Pregnancy
20. Race: strokes more common in black Americans than whites
21. Raised serum fibrinogen levels
22. Sex: strokes more common in men than in women
23. Sleep related disorders: snoring and sleep apnea
24. Smoking
25. Transient ischemic attacks

How is a stroke diagnosed?

It's hard for a lay person to know whether or not someone is actually experiencing the first symptoms of a stroke, but Jain says it's also hard for a physician to diagnose. There are so many possible variations in the initial presenting symptoms:

It is essential that a stroke patient be clinically examined (symptoms) as well as by laboratory tests. Treatment of an acute ischemic stroke is critical because there is a short window of opportunity to prevent or limit irreversible damage to the brain.

Jain and the American Stroke Association agree that:

> *The ideal place for a patient is a stroke center. If this is not available, a major general hospital with neurological service would be adequate.*

He admits these goals may be extremely difficult to attain, and concludes by saying patients should be treated on an emergency basis within an hour of occurrence.

Jain defines the current objectives of acute stroke therapy as:

1. Reduce the mortality rate to below 20 percent
2. Restoration of normal blood flow
   a. Thrombolysis of blood flow obstructing cerebral arteries
   b. Surgical procedures such as endarterectomy
3. Cerebral protection against the effects of ischemia
   a. Hyperbaric oxygen
   b. Neuroprotectives
4. Supportive medical care
   a. Maintenance of airway and oxygenation
   b. Management of concomitant diseases such as heart disease and hypertension
5. Maintenance of fluid and electrolyte balance
   a. Prevention of complications such as aspiration phenomena
6. Preservation of life and management of systemic effects of stroke

7. Neurologic intensive care
   a. Monitoring of increased intracranial pressure
   b. Management of neurological complications, e.g., cerebral edema and seizures
8. Prevention of disease extension and recurrence
   a. Anticoagulation/antiplatelet therapy
   b. Risk factor management
9. Rehabilitation: To enable 70 percent of the stroke survivors to live independently three months after stroke.

Jain's advice for the protocol or procedure that should be followed by every emergency room physician is as follows:

The symptoms can vary depending on where the infarcted artery is located and which cranial nerves or sensory pathways are involved. Trained and experienced ambulance attendants can recognize stroke in a fair percentage of patients. Supplementary oxygen is usually given in the ambulance and an intravenous line established.

In some countries, blood pressure is regularly checked. Ambulance personnel notify the emergency medical facility to have necessary personnel and equipment available, including an emergency CT scan and alerting the emergency physician to the possibility that the patient may be a candidate for tPA therapy.

In the emergency department of the hospital, the patient's airway and circulation is checked on arrival and supplemental oxygen and intravenous saline or Ringer solution is started.

Dr. Jain says supplementary oxygen should be routinely administered to a possible stroke patient, both in the ambulance and in the hospital, but the American Stroke Association's protocol actually discourages the use of oxygen. The ASA's exact words on their website in 2004 were:

> *Maintaining adequate tissue oxygenation is an important component of emergent management. Hypoxia results in anaerobic metabolism and depletion of energy stores that can increase the extent of brain injury and worsen outcome...No data establish the benefit of supplementary oxygen and there is no reason to routinely administer this therapy...It's role in the general treatment of acute ischemic stroke has not been adequately tested.*

I continue to ask the question: How can our publicly-supported American experts dare to say the role of oxygen still "has not been tested," when their own stroke definition tells us, *"adequate tissue oxygenation is an important component of emergent management,"* and they add, *"Hypoxia can increase the extent of brain damage"*?

Jain also recommends getting an eyewitness account of the onset of a stroke because the patient's memory may not be reliable. He stresses the importance of learning the time and symptoms of the onset, and says neurological dysfunction should be recorded, and an examination repeated to see

135

whether the stroke is recovering, stable, or increasing. In 1996, he laid out the management protocols for treating an acute stroke:

1. Medical therapies:
   a. Thrombolytic therapy
   b. Anticoagulant therapy
   c. Antiplatelet agents
   d. Hemorrheological agents: Trental
   e. Drugs for reduction of cerebral edema
   f. Management of hypotension
   g. Complementary medical therapies: herbs and acupuncture
2. Hyperbaric oxygen
3. Management of concomitant disorders
   a. Antihypertensive medications
   b. Drugs for cardiac disorders
4. Surgical therapies
   a. Evaluation of intracerebral hematomas
   b. Decompressive craniotomy
   c. Carotid endartectomy
   d. Embolectomy
   e. Transluminal angioplasty
   f. Surgical procedures for revascularization
5. Start of rehabilitation

There are many available tools for acute stroke treatment as shown here. The medical world is *NOT* limited to tPA, with its six percent recovery record.

Role of Oxygen

The human brain requires between 500 and 600 milliliters of oxygen per minute. That's 25 percent of the body's total oxygen consumption. If the flow is completely blocked, neuronal metabolism will be damaged within six seconds. Activity will cease after two minutes. At five minutes, brain tissues begin to die. Depending on the degree of oxygen blockage, these changes are reversible for up to a few hours, and some recovery of function can take place after days, weeks, months, or even years. However, Jain writes:

> ...*The traditional concept of infarction, that the brain tissue dies after a shortage of blood and oxygen lasting more than a few minutes, is no longer valid. The interruption of blood flow is seldom total and a drop in cerebral blood flow to as low as 50% can maintain function.*

This information helped me answer some of my questions. Jain gives the following time sequence for a stroke:

1. Transient ischemic attacks (TIA)	Minutes to 24 hours
2. Reversible ischemic neurological deficit (RIND)	Hours
3. Prolonged reversible ischemic neurological deficit (PRIND) (stroke in evolution)	Days
4. Brain infarction with fixed neurological deficit (completed stroke)	Hours to months

5. Chronic post-stroke stage

More than
one year
after onset

Does a stroke happen slowly or "all at once"? Is treatment possible after more than those first three hours? How long does the "acute" phase last? I now understand more of what's going on inside a brain during those minutes, hours, or days. Jain reminds his readers that "although ischemia is a circulatory disorder, the impact is determined by neurological changes at the subcellular level."

> *Within the central area of impact, a blood flow rate of 10 ml/g/minute or less creates a rise of extracellular K, drop in ADP, increase of lactate and intracellular acidosis.*
>
> *At the boundary of the infarction, with a blood flow rate of 0.10 to 0.15 ml/g/minute, we find an extinction of neuronal electricity, and a limited rise of extracellular K.*
>
> *In the collateral zone, at a greater rate than 0.15 ml/g/minute, we find hyperemia with no disturbed metabolism.*
>
> *...These biochemical changes, known as excitotoxic substances, have been measured in experimental laboratory animals. Researchers have found damagingly high levels of glutamate and other amino acids to be a dominant factor in brain tissue injuries. Current research in biopharmaceutical firms is based on ways to prevent this damage.*

Jain delves more deeply into neurological damage at the molecular level, telling us what has been learned about those genes that regulate growth and differentiation, about heat-shock proteins, the inflammatory-immunologic reactions of ischemia, DNA damage, neurotrophic factors, and neuronal damage. You'll find a broad-brush look in Chapter 9 at the breakthroughs he and others predict may be possible in the future for brain repair and reconstruction.

Jain also discusses free radicals, explaining that they can cause protein oxidation, DNA destruction, increased intracellular calcium, activation of damaging proteases and nucleases, and peroxidation of cellular membrane lipids. Damaged cells lead to the formation of prostaglandins, interferons, free radicals, and other substances; too much of anything can be devastating.

My daughter explained the free radical problem to me with this example: "Imagine a bomb going off in the engine room of a cruise ship, right next to the sewage system. First the toilets all jam up, then they start flooding the engine room. Now imagine the crew and all the passengers suddenly being ordered to each carry a bucket down to the disaster area, fill their bucket with the muck, haul it up to the deck, dump it overboard, and return for more until the mess is all cleared away." She continued, "If you think of canisters of fire extinguishers filled with fire-retardant foam as being comparable to the body's antioxidant defense system, you can see how the mess created by the body's defense system can become part of the problem."

Conventional doctors are taught that administering additional oxygen increases oxidative stress. It is this bit of incorrect knowledge that has led many doctors to dismiss the usefulness of pressurized oxygen. The neurologist, however, says there is *NO* valid evidence that oxygen is harmful to a patient having a stroke. This is one situation where a little bit of doctor knowledge may be dangerous to the patient.

This brings us to reperfusion, or the problems that sometimes arise when the flow of blood is too suddenly restored. The blockage may have cleared spontaneously, may been dissolved by tPA, or by surgery to clear an artery. With oxygen once again available, cell metabolism is restored and free radicals can be cleared from the bloodstream. But, Jain warns, a too-sudden surge of blood has sometimes caused more damage to fragile, already-injured tissues, upset the calcium balance, and created a fresh flood of free radicals, leukocyte-mediated injuries, and hyper-cholesterolemia. In other words, he warns that surgical removal of the clot has sometimes created additional stroke damage. Pressurized oxygen can avoid this damage by providing a gradual increase of oxygen in the blood.

This is what the brain can do to heal itself:

It is well recognized that spontaneous, often dramatic improvement occurs in patients with acute ischemic stroke. About one-fourth...show improvement by one hour, and nearly half show some improvement by six hours. Few of these patients, however, show complete motor recovery. Ninety percent remain improved on long-term follow-up, indicating that improvement during the first 48 hours after ischemic stroke is a predictor of favorable long-term outcome.

When I read this I remembered how "things" had slowly "come back" in the days and weeks following my stroke. My right hand, which had been curled into a fist and almost useless, began slowly "coming back to life" while I was in the nursing/rehab facility. During those two weeks, I progressed from being absolutely unable to "walk" the fingers of my right hand up even two "steps" on a hand-flexibility tool that was hanging on the wall, no matter how hard I tried. One triumphant morning I could "run" my fingers nimbly up the ladder. And my walking improved, from being limited to a wheelchair, to haltingly limping the length of a corridor.

Here is Jain's description of the brain's methods for replacing the "wiring" of damaged tissues:

1. Presence of collateral blood supply. The degree of motor improvement offers opportunities for secondary perifocal neuronal reorganization. Mapping of the extent of the penumbra enables prediction for potential of recovery.
2. Regression of cerebral edema.
3. Volume of penumbra that escapes infarction offers opportunities for secondary perifocal neuronal reorganization. Mapping of the extent of the penumbra enables prediction for potential of recovery.
4. There is considerable scope for functional plasticity in the adult human cerebral cortex.

Cortical reorganization is associated with functional recovery in experimental and human stroke. Retraining after stroke can extend cortical representation of the infarcted area and improve skilled motor performance, and correlates with cerebral blood flow values in the undamaged cortex of the opposite cerebral hemisphere.

Jain further explains that cerebral energy metabolism is essential to the recovery of brain function, and that it depends on restoring blood flow, but warns:

> Post ischemic resynthesis is limited. The recovery process is far more complex than the simple process of reversal of ischemia by revascularization.

He continues:

> The size of the penumbra zone is an important factor in regaining brain function. Sometimes it is difficult to distinguish between the area blasted by the infarction and those cells in the penumbra that still have a potential for recovery.

I realized this explained Dr. Neubauer's use of a SPECT scan before and after each HBO treatment. A SPECT scan can actually measure any increase in the flow of blood in the penumbra, thus identifying the living, but lethargic, brain cells.

Note: If you, or someone you care about has had a stroke and is getting better—don't relax too soon.

The patient may not be out of the woods yet. Jain lists the following complications that have been reported in the literature. According to a 1998 study, 95 percent of stroke survivors had at least one of these complications during the first week—a decrease in consciousness or increase of neurological deficits. Sometimes the cause was a fresh hemorrhage at the site of the infarct. Other patients have had such metabolic disturbances as hypoglycemia or hyponatremia, or been adversely affected by drugs. He lists some of these complications:

1. Progressive neurological deficits
2. Cerebral edema with transtenorial herniations
3. Extension of infarction or appearance of a new infarct
4. Hemorrhagic transformation of infarct
5. Seizures

Now that I'd seen Dr. Jain's list of "what could have happened," I could understand why I'd been kept in the hospital for observation during the week after my "minor" stroke. I was unnaturally drowsy—probably the result of all that swelling going on in my brain, and things have been known to go from bad to worse for a few unfortunate stroke victims.

What hope is there for recovery after a stroke? What research is in the works? What are today's dollar-oriented biopharmaceutical firms investigating in their efforts to make a buck or two?

Jain lists the following areas of current interest:

1. Redefinition of thrombolitic therapy (tPA)
2. Value of early intravenous heparin
     following ischemic stroke
3. Value of antiplatelet therapy given during
     the first six hours after stroke onset
4. Neuroprotective therapy for acute stroke
5. Value of hyperbaric oxygenation in acute
     ischemic stroke
6. Value of hypothermia in acute ischemic stroke
7. Combination of various therapies

He includes more than one hundred patentable compounds that were in various stages of development in 1997. These were:

1. Thrombolytics
2. Anticoagulants
3. Defibrinogenating agents
4. Agents to improve hemorrheology
5. Neuroprotectives
     a. Adenosine analogs
     b. Anti-inflammatory agents
     c. Apoptosis inhibitors
     1. Calpain inhibitors
     2. Cycloheximidine
     d. Ion Channel modulators
     1. Ca++ channel blockers
     2. Na++ channel blockers
6. NMDA antagonists
     a. NMDA receptor antagonists—competitive
        and non-competitive

     b. AMPA antagonists
     c. Glycine site antagonists
  7. Non-NMDA excitatory amino acid
     antagonists
     a. 5-HT agonist
     b. GABA agonists
     c. Opioid receptor antagonists
  8. Nitric oxide scavengers
  9. Free radical scavengers
10. Drugs counteracting lactate neurotoxicity
11. Agents for regeneration and repair
     a. Neurotropic factors
     b. Nootropic agents
     c. Phosphotidylcholine synthesis
12. Hormonal modulators of cerebral ischemia
13. Anti-edema agents
14. Antihypoxic agents
15. Miscellaneous agents
16. Oxygen carriers
17. Gene therapy

When I read the list, it suggested a reason why the medical world has turned its back on oxygen. Oxygen is just too cheap and too readily available. It's probably those potential dollars that are keeping today's scientists (and their CEOs) searching for a "magic bullet" for oxygen-deprived brains. Jain finishes this portion of his "Stroke" chapter by saying:

> *With so many choices available for experimental therapies for stroke, many combination therapies are being considered.*

He suggests that doctors use a combination of available thrombolytics and neuroprotectives. He states that they can be administered simultaneously to address different problems. He looks at the use of thrombolytics and HBO, saying HBO can protect the brain against ischemia/hypoxia during the first hours while the patient is being transported and examined, before being given thrombolitic therapy. This would give the medical community the best of both worlds— control of the edema, allowing physicians additional time to administer one or more of those commercial new drugs.

9

THE CHRONIC STROKE

Portions of this chapter, like Chapter 8, are filled with medical terminology, but all of it is critical to understanding the depths of strokes.

I've separated K.K. Jain's work into two separate chapters because the beneficial effects of HBO on each phase of a stroke are very different. As you've seen, during the acute phase, while brain cells are being progressively destroyed, additional oxygen can reduce swollen blood vessels and deliver oxygen molecules to starving cells. In other words, oxygen can rescue those endangered brain cells. But after the stroke has stabilized, oxygen's role is quite different.

What are the long-term effects of a stroke? Paralyzed muscles (muscles that refuse to move on command) are among the many disabilities that a brain injury causes. If you've ever had the electricity go off during a storm, you'll understand what this means. Power is available at the source. But you click the light switch and nothing happens. There's been a break in the delivery line.

In a strange sort of way, HBO's role in chronic stroke recovery is like the story of Sleeping Beauty. Our hero Prince Oxygen has to fight his way through a tangled web of chronically swollen blood vessels before he can awaken "sleeping" brain cells. But that's not the "happily ever after" end of the story. Before those brain cells can "wake up" permanently, our prince must trigger the growth of new capillaries, and that takes time. This takes lots of time.

In many medical centers, "chronic" means you've had all the physical therapy you're going to get, and the doctors have said you've recovered as much of your lost functions as you ever will. At least that was the medical attitude toward me and most of the other stroke victims I met.

Let's see what Jain has to tell us about the "chronic" stage:

> The neuronal structure can be preserved with cerebral blood flow as low as 15%–20% of normal. Between the zones of infarction and normal brain tissue is a third zone referred to as the "penumbra," containing the so-called dormant or "idling" neurons. These neurons are nonfunctional but anatomically intact and can be revived. The presence of viable brain tissue in the penumbra explains why the clinical presentation of a completed stroke is a rather poor predictor of the outcome. A trickle of blood flow is maintained in the penumbra zone, which is hypoxic. It can be presumed that the critical parameter for cellular function is oxygen availability rather than blood flow.

Those words, "the presence of viable brain tissue," echoed in my head as I scoured the Internet.

The recovery time scale, Jain says, is both variable and controversial. Most motor recovery occurs during the first three months, although some functional recovery can be regained in the next six months or even as long as a year after the stroke.

Here's how Jain describes the recovery of lost functions:

1. Unmasking or release from inhibition of previously non-functioning pathways.
2. Synaptic sprouting and formation of new dendritic connections for pathways for transmission of neural messages.

This neural unmasking, he says, is the basis for the growing field of neuroplasticity, a term describing the body's ability to regrow its own neural structures.

Jain lists the factors influencing stroke-recovery:

1. Neurological status of the patient
   a. prior to stroke
   b. immediately following stroke
2. Age
3. Type of stroke
4. Location of lesion in the cerebral arteries
5. Risk factors of stroke
6. Treatment of stroke

That information helped to explain the plateau I was stuck on. My body has always swelled when any part is injured. A sprained ankle meant I was in for a swollen foot and lower leg. A bruised finger meant a swollen hand. Why was I surprised because my 77-year-old brain had swelled after it was injured?

Jain says, "the appearance of neurological sequelae may be extensions of the damage that arose during the acute stage of a stroke." These sequelae are important, but are not always detected when the stroke has stabilized.

1. Persistence of neurological deficits
2. Epilepsy
3. Spasticity
4. Central pain syndrome
5. Neuro-psychological disturbances
    a. Memory disturbances
    b. Intellectual and cognitive impairment
    c. Dementia
    d. Depression
    e. Pseudo-depressive manifestations
    f. Anxiety
    g. Apathy
    h. Pathological laughing and crying
    j. Mania

Perhaps I ought to be happy, not angry and frustrated, that I've been left with only three of the above: the persistence of neurological defects in one arm and a leg, moderate spasticity, and short-term memories that I can't always depend on, but I am frustrated because maybe I could be much better.

Here's an amazing stroke recovery story I found on the Internet, written March 1, 2001, about a severe hemorrhagic stroke. The writer said he was a retired high-ranking Naval officer who had seen the effectiveness of HBO for stroke treatment.

This man and his wife had been on a camping vacation when she had a stroke. He immediately recognized the symptoms, and within two hours had her in the nearest hospital, only fifteen miles away, where she was given tPA, which caused massive bleeding. Her husband asked that she be treated with hyperbaric oxygen while she was still in the emergency room because he'd seen oxygen used effectively in the Navy for treating a stroke. The attending physician refused, saying, "He'd never heard of it."

His wife's condition deteriorated rapidly, so he had her transferred to a hospital in Virginia where the physicians promised "more aggressive treatment." This hospital actually had a hyperbaric chamber available, but the director refused to allow the woman to be treated, insisting that HBO for neurological disorders was only "experimental" and not "scientifically proven."

When I read this statement, I thought, "What did the HBO director have to lose?" Why wouldn't he at least make the scorned "experimental" or "off label" treatment available after the naval officer assured the director that he would take full responsibility and pay all charges? Instead, the chamber director refused to allow her inside "his" chamber.

I'll let the writer tell you what happened next:

After she stabilized, my wife spent the next fifteen months in a vegetative state in a well-respected rehabilitation center. Despite physical therapy (PT) and occupational therapy (OT), her right arm and leg remained flaccid. I continued asking that she be given HBOT, a treatment I'd seen used effectively for strokes in the Navy. Eventually, the director of the rehab facility agreed to "allow" me to take my wife to a nearby free-standing HBOT clinic if I could get a release from Medicaid. Ninety-seven HBOT treatments later, my wife had regained fifty percent mobility and at least as much cognitive strength. At that point she plateaued, in spite of continuing her physical and occupational therapy. Six months later she was given forty-three additional HBOT treatments and once again improved in both mobility and cognitive strength. Today she is able to walk short distances while maintaining her balance. Her cognitive strength (understanding) continues to improve. She has not yet regained speech but she gives directions through gestures and occasionally says a word or two. With continued therapy, she is expected to recover her speech.

I think you'll agree, this was a "worst case" scenario—a severe hemorrhage leaving the victim unable to speak or walk and a fifteen-month delay before oxygen therapy was started. A severe bleed and tPA, the treatment that had been administered, had caused further massive damage. She was denied an available treatment that MIGHT have helped. Partial recovery fifteen months later, after being treated with pressurized oxygen. If ever HBO was put to the test, this was such a test.

I wonder how many stroke victims today are stuck in nursing homes, vegetating, because they haven't been treated with pressurized oxygen, a safe therapy that could restore some of their still-living but "dormant" neurons.

Jain notes the scarcity of stroke recovery therapies:

"In contrast to the tremendous efforts being made in the management of acute stroke, little is done for the patient in the chronic post-stroke stage. Most of these patients have been discharged to home, and very few receive regular physical therapy. Physicians are seldom interested in these post-stroke patients who are considered to have fixed neurological deficits due to irreversible brain damage...However, conventional and sometimes innovative efforts have been made with patients in the chronic post-stroke stage for the management of spasticity, improvement of motor deficits, and treatment of dementia.

Jain discusses spasticity (rigid muscles) in detail, saying spasticity is the most troublesome complication of stroke and a major obstacle to physical rehabilitation. He lists the currently available treatments for spasticity management:

1. Physical medicine: heat, cold, vibration, electrical stimulation
2. Physical therapy: splints, positioning of patients, spasm-inhibiting exercises, slow and prolonged stretching
3. Drugs: dantrolene, baclofen, diazepam, phenylation plus chlorpromazine
4. Surgery:
    a. Orthopedic: lengthening, sectioning, release and transposition of tendons
    b. Neurosurgical: Intramuscular neurolysis and rhizotomy, spinal cord stimulation, intrathecal baclofen, tizanadine

I've included the neurologist's list of current medical strategies for improving damaged motor functions. If you or someone you know is having a recovery problem, you might find a new or different drug or treatment here, one that your physician hasn't considered, but, in the words of our pharmaceutical advertising gurus, "First, ask your doctor."

Drugs:

1. ACH chlorhydrate
2. Amphetamine
3. Apomorphine
4. Caffeine
5. Carbaminol choline
6. Fluoxetine
7. GM, gangliosides
8. Levadopa
9. Neostigmine
10. Norepinephrine
11. Phenylpropanolamine
12. Yohimbine
13. Promotion of neural regeneration and enhancement of synaptic plasticity
14. Surgical procedures
    a. Cerebral revascularization
    b. Neural transplantation

Of all the drugs studied in animal experiments, Jain says amphetamine was the most consistently reported to have accelerated the recovery of function. Explaining the effectiveness of the drug, he says amphetamines have a variety of effects on brain neurons. He describes a significant interaction in the central nervous system between acetylcholine and norepinepherine via the alpha-l receptors, modulating the direct release of acetylcholine from the cerebral cortex. This release is also mediated by gamma amino butyric acid, using the connections between the locus coeruleus, on the floor of the fourth ventricle, and the cholinergic cells in the septum, hippocampus, and cerebral cortex.

He adds these words for physicians who may be reluctant to prescribe amphetamine for their patients: "Intraventricular infusions of norepinepherine appear to mimic the amphetamine effect in laboratory animals, but dopamine infusions had no effect on laboratory animals. Amphetamine appears to promote the growth of alternate circuits—an advantage for stroke recovery. A double-blind human pilot study in 1998 reported that amphetamine combined with physical therapy had measurably aided the recovery of motor function in stroke patients," and he concludes, "Norepinepherine release may be the integral controlling factor in recovering motor function after stroke."

However, Jain warns of this drug:

1. Amphetamine can aggravate rather than improve spasticity.
2. It is contraindicated in several conditions, including hypertension, which is frequent in stroke patients.
3. It is habit-forming and has other undesirable side effects.

Constraint-Induced Therapy

A new technique designed to coax the brain into reorganizing itself has recently made headlines. In a paper published in July, 1999, in the *Journal of Rehabilitation Research and Development,* Dr. Edward Taub, a psychologist at the University of Alabama in Birmingham, said he believes the value of massive repetitive therapy movements after stroke has not been fully tested.

Taub's theory grows out of his experiments with monkeys. A group of monkeys were given surgical injuries. The control animals were allowed to recover when and as they were able. In primates, healing takes from two to six months after a cerebrovascular injury. At first, all the animals failed when they attempted to swing, jump, or even hold food firmly with the affected limb. As a result of these failures, the monkeys learned to ignore the "useless" limb and used only the remaining three. In some of the treated monkeys, the non-affected forelimb was immobilized while the animal was still surgically anesthetized, forcing the monkey to use the injured forelimb. Three months later, after the restraint was removed, they were able to use the limb that had been immobilized, while the monkeys whose non-affected limb had not been restrained had "learned" they couldn't trust the affected one, and still used only the other three limbs.

I can't help but question Taub's theory. It's true that after a stroke, when a patient discovers an arm or a hand "won't work," he will stop trying to use it. That arm or hand *will not* work until the blocked electrical impulses are restored or new neural connections have been built.

156

The last fifty years have brought technical improvements that allow researchers to actually measure brain activity. Taub was interested in the specific area of the brain that controls movements of the thumb and wrist. His group was able to measure the electrical activity representing rewiring in the human brain as a result of massive amounts of aggressive, controlled physical therapy. It was his belief that any permanent increase of movement in a stroke-damaged arm or hand would involve two ideas:

(1) The patient would learn that the wrist or hand *could* now be used; that depending on the non-affected limb was no longer necessary.
(2) Sustained and repeated practice would increase the number of brain cells on the non-involved side, making any improvements permanent.

For his first experiment, twenty-five men and women, post-stroke at least one year, had their brains mapped by transcranial magnetic stimulation (TMS) to measure the size of the brain area controlling movements before treatment. Thirteen of the patients had their good arm tied down (secured in a splint and sling) for fourteen consecutive days. On ten of these days they were given six hours of supervised task practice using only the free (affected) arm: eating lunch, throwing a ball, playing dominoes, Chinese checkers or card games, writing, pushing a broom, or working with manipulation test equipment, interspersed with one hour rest periods. These thirteen spent eight days in the rehabilitation laboratory, working six hours a day at attempting small grasping and moving movements. At the end of two weeks, they had regained three-quarters of the normal use of their paralyzed arms.

The control subjects were told that they *could* move the affected limb "if they wanted to," and were given a series of passive movement exercises to be done in the treatment center and at home. When tested after two weeks, the control group showed no change, but the treatment group had a very large increase in real-world arm and hand use. Two years later, the treated group showed a further small increase, while the control group showed either no change or a decline in arm use.

Later constraint-therapy experiments have concentrated on a patient's individual motor deficits, with therapists helping a patient to carry out some parts of a movement sequence when the patient was not able to complete the movement. Praise was generous for small improvements.

In this second experiment, the control group patients were told they were to evaluate the duration and intensity of therapist-patient sessions, and the duration and intensity of therapeutic activities. They were given a general fitness program of strength, balance, and stamina exercises; they played games to stimulate their cognitive activity, and practiced relaxation skills for ten days.

At the end of the sessions, the constraint therapy group displayed a significant increase in motor abilities and in real-world arm use. The control group did not.

Other groups have suggested additional techniques for overcoming learned nonuse, including wearing a padded half-glove on the "good" arm (for the safety of patients with balance problems), intensive physical therapy, aquatic therapy, neurophysiological facilitation, and task practices that involve using the problem arm for ten consecutive days. All groups showed a large increase in the use of the affected arm in real-life situations.

The Taub group reports that other laboratories in the United States, Germany, and Sweden have replicated their findings. They conclude that it is repetitive practice, not the use of a sling or glove, that has achieved good results. There was little or no gain without concentrated, repetitive practice of a movement.

Recent examinations using TMS have revealed that in the unused, affected area of the brain, the cellular network will shrink, sometimes as much as seventy percent. After intensive constraint-induced therapy, the active brain area has been found to have nearly doubled.

According to a June 2, 2000, *New York Times* story by Sandra Blakeslee, approximately two hundred and fifty patients have been given constraint-induced therapy in the United States and at the Freidrich Schiller University of Jena, Germany. Many have regained nearly full use of paralyzed limbs through this intensive therapy.

Nancy Shute of *U.S. News and World Reports* wrote on June 26, 2000, "mounting evidence suggests that the adult brain is capable of regeneration—a feat long thought impossible. Researchers are learning that intensive therapy actually promotes new connections in the brain, months, or even decades, after a disabling stroke." She goes on to report that the Massachusetts Institute of Technology has invented a robot that can "play therapist," spending hours a day with a stroke patient, gauging and adjusting itself to the patient's strength while helping him or her to play "connect the dots." She quotes a physical therapy professor as saying, "Constraint-induced therapy is so simple that people can do it on their own." In the words of one stroke patient attemping home treatment, "It takes ten thousand repetitions of the same movement, and that's a lot."

A former constraint-induced therapy patient suggests, "Find simple exercises that you can do with your affected side. Repeat them every day for an hour. Flip dominoes, play connect four, pick up cans of vegetables, stack checkers, take a spoon and use a bowl full of beans, transfer a spoonful at a time into another bowl, ring toss, stack plastic cups, use key to open car door. Remember, doing it once or twice doesn't help. Repetition is the key."

Now for a look at hyperbaric oxygenation.

Dr. Jain lists eleven standard "acute" uses for oxygen that physicians should be aware of, fifty-seven "chronic," and eleven that were still called *exploratory* in 1997, when the third edition of his text was published. The list has continued to grow as physicians throughout the world have reported on ailments they have successfully treated with HBO.

Hyperbaric oxygen can play an important role in cerebral ischemia, the neurologist says, reminding his readers of the greater resistance to blood flow in capillaries less than 1.5mm in diameter. In these tiny blood vessels, the red blood cells are squeezed into a column rather than flowing randomly, but even during a momentary slowing or clumping of cells, plasma can still seep around the obstacle.

This is Jain's description of hyperbaric oxygen's activity:

1. Oxygen dissolved in plasma under pressure can nourish tissues even in the absence of red blood cells.
2. Oxygen can diffuse extravascularly, facilitated by the difference between the high oxygen tension in the patent capillaries and the low tension in the occluded ones. The effectiveness of this mechanism depends on the abundance of capillaries in the tissues. Because the brain is a very vascular tissue, the mechanism can provide for the oxygenation of the tissues after vascular occlusion.
3. The supply of oxygen to the tissues can be facilitated by decreasing the viscosity of the blood and reducing platelet aggregation and increasing red blood cell deformability.
4. By its vasoconstricting action, HBO relieves brain edema, counteracting the vasodilation of the capillaries in the hypoxic tissues and reducing the extravasation of fluid.
5. HBO also reduces the swelling of the neurons by improving their metabolism.
6. By improving oxygenation of the penumbra that surrounds the zone of total ischemia, HBO prevents glycolysis and subsequent intracellular lactic acidosis, and maintains cerebral metabolism in an otherwise compromised area.

Jain's text, along with hyperbaric physicians offering HBO as an "after-stroke" treatment, fails to mention "regression." What happens inside a chronically swollen brain when the supplemental oxygen is withdrawn? In my opinion, there is good reason to emphasize the need for giving a stroke patient supplemental oxygen during the acute phase. We all know it's much faster and easier to heal a bruise than to repair a broken bone.

Current Research

Today's researchers have investigated chronic stroke by artificially creating stroke damage in animals.

In the laboratory, the effects of hypoxia can be studied under controlled conditions. Rats are the most popular subjects for these experiments because the blood vessels in a rat's brain closely resemble those in a human. And, Jain adds, using rats, rather than dogs, cats, or monkeys is less expensive and less objectionable to the animal rights movement.

The standard (scientifically approved) model of focal ischemia has been to surgically block an artery, usually the middle cerebral artery, because the procedure can be reliably reproduced by other researchers in other laboratories. This kind of experiment has given biopharmaceutical firms vital information in their efforts to create neuroprotectants. Microscopically examining a slide of the damaged brain tissue is the usual way of evaluating a drug's effectiveness, or the results can be measured in living animals by using MRI (magnetic resonance imaging). Animal models may not precisely mimic the human stroke, but a new drug's effect on injured brain cells can be reliably measured.

Today's electronic wizards have invented a number of ingenious new tools that allow the researchers to actually "watch" what goes on inside a living brain. SPECT (single photon emission computerized tomography) scans can accurately measure "where" and "how much" electrical and/or metabolic activity is taking place in a living brain. Dr. Neubauer reports using a SPECT scan before and after each HBO treatment to measure the extent and/or increase of brain metabolism. He states that the ischemic penumbra is pretty much in place four to six hours after a clot has formed in the brain, although it may take as long as eighteen hours before the swelling stabilizes.

I asked the well-known hyperbaric physician, Dr. Philip B. James of Edinburgh, Scotland, how stroke patients in Great Britain are treated to prevent this devastating secondary damage.

His reply:

There is a way to prevent both primary and secondary damage by using surgery in combination with oxygen. In acute stroke, PET imaging has shown that the ischemic penumbra continues to change for at least 18 hours. Using oxygen in addition to surgery, the window for avoiding primary damage can be extended far beyond 4 hours.

This is when I first learned about stents (coiled wires), shunts (tubes), and sophisticated new surgical techniques to prop open a blocked artery.

But surgery means hospitals and expert neurological surgeons, so HBO isn't the entire answer.

I was very depressed when I went to sleep that night. I thought maybe the American Stroke Association was right. There may be no practical way, in the geographically sprawling United States, to prevent serious, lasting damage.

But something in this jigsaw puzzle didn't fit.

In Dr. James' letter that had so discouraged me, he'd added:

> *If you asked me if I would have HBOT if I had a completed stroke—the answer is YES, because it may offer some improvement in my quality of life and it is safe. Loss of function in the brain can be due either to tissue swelling, which IS REVERSIBLE, or tissue destruction, which IS NOT...We all know that measurable tissue edema (swelling) can persist elsewhere in the body for many years. We see this chronic swelling in arthritic joints. Now SPECT imaging has shown us that measurable tissue edema may persist in the brain for many years.*

That was when I finally realized that Dr. Neubauer had been discussing a "chronic" or "completed" stroke when he'd written:

> *Activation of those neurons explains why patients can show improvement when HBOT is administered*

years after a stroke occurs—in some cases, up to thirteen years later...Out of 79 patients, treated from five months to ten years after their strokes, 65 percent reported improvement in their quality of life.

I Decide to 'Go for It'

I was convinced that **something COULD be done to bring my brain back to life.** The emergency room doctor had said, "I'd only had a minor stroke," and my regular doctor had congratulated me, calling me, "So lucky." Maybe my doctor was right. I was sure that many of my reluctant brain cells were still alive, because they worked in the morning but "conked" out in the afternoon when I was tired. They were "intermittent," and intermittent means on-again-off-again. Sometimes awake, sometimes asleep. I was sure they just needed a push to get them working again.

In the words of one hyperbaric scientist:

In the stabilized stroke the main function of pressurized oxygen is the rebuilding of capillaries, relieving the hypoxia, reducing brain edema or swelling, restoring the integrity of the damaged cell membranes, and neutralizing the toxic waste products."

I thought, that's exactly what I need. Still, I couldn't help wondering...So many of the medical experts I'd found on the Internet had either ignored or scoffed at hyperbaric oxygen. One physician had scornfully tagged it "a treatment in search of a disease." Could those reported improvements possibly be a simple placebo effect? Or just temporary?

I was reassured by a posting from Dr. Volpe, a pediatric neurologist who works primarily with cerebral palsy children. He had written in the *Annals of Neurology* (17(3):287–96, 1985):

> *Is Hyperbaric Oxygen permanent? Yes, absolutely. HBOT is also used for burns, gangrene, crush injuries, and wound healing, etc. Have you ever heard of a 3rd degree burn suddenly recurring 5 years after it was healed? No, of course not. Pressurized oxygen therapy (HBOT) essentially works by forcing the growth of new capillary systems into damaged tissue. Once circulation is restored, function is restored and healing occurs.*
>
> *The same restoration of function after circulation restoration has also happened to you and me. How many times have you awakened in the middle of the night only to discover that your arm has "fallen asleep" because you slept on it funny and cut off the circulation? That arm doesn't work. You don't have feeling or movement in that arm until circulation is restored.*

A final quote from the Internet, 14 Nov. 1999:

> *Does anyone seriously dispute that the correction of a serious oxygen deficiency should be the first objective of any physician/surgeon...when a brain crying out for oxygen, with a few exceptions, goes untreated?*

Excited by the thought of reviving my dozing brain, I cruised the Internet looking for a local HBO facility, but Oregon, the state where we live, listed **none.** Not one single hyperbaric chamber in the entire state. This was very discouraging, as we'd retired to Oregon because it was "so progressive."

However, in the year 1999, I found thirteen free-standing facilities listed in California. One was in Chico, a northern California town where my youngest daughter lived, only a five-hour drive away.

Five *hours* is a comfortable drive for a family visit, but it would be useless in a medical emergency, when minutes can cost a life.

But that wasn't my problem; I was now a stable, chronic stroke survivor. I called the director of the Chico facility. He recommended forty treatments, two a day, five days a week for a month. He explained, "You say you had your stroke two years ago. Forty treatments is the standard suggested treatment for chronic, stabilized strokes." He offered to give me the telephone number of a caregiver who was very enthusiastic over her husband's partial recovery, saying, "She could tell me about the changes she had seen." He would need a prescription from my doctor, and warned me that he could not **guarantee** any improvement.

I was sure that many of my non-functioning brain cells were still alive because of that on-again, off-again performance that depended on the time of day and whether I was fatigued or rested. I was willing to try anything that might improve my quality of life, but a whole month is a long time for a handicapped old lady and her 84-year-old, slow-moving husband to live with an adult daughter and her active family.

We wondered if we could manage the stairs in her home, because she lives is a two-story house with all the bedrooms upstairs. Could we climb those stairs on a daily basis?

Next I talked with my primary care doctor because the Chico clinic required a physician's permission. He is a moderately young man, alert to the latest medical trends and a graduate of a highly respected medical school. His reply when I asked him about HBO was, "Sorry. I don't know anything about it." I showed him some of my printouts from the Internet and he agreed to write a prescription, BUT on condition that I **not** ask my health insurance to pay for it. His explanation was that, "The paperwork demanded by our insurance provider is just too time-consuming, and they would deny it anyway."

The forty sessions would cost us $95 each. We aren't wealthy, but my husband and I had agreed it would be worth it if HBO helped me regain even a part of my lost quality of life.

Here's the diary I kept, to record one miraculous recovery after another.

10

THE BIG ADVENTURE

Monday, November 1, 1999: This is it. Day one. What is breathing pressurized oxygen going to be like? I've read everything I could get my hands on about HBO, but reading about something isn't the same as doing it.

The Chico Hyperbaric Center is located in a newish storefront building on the southern edge of this rapidly growing California town. This is a "freestanding" hyperbaric clinic, not part of a hospital complex. It's much more efficient and far less expensive to operate a hyperbaric clinic as a separate facility, under the supervision of well-trained hyperbaric therapists and technicians, when the facility is used primarily, as this one is, for treating chronic ailments.

The story behind the Chico clinic is interesting.

In 1997, Dr. Mitchell Hoggard, a pharmacist (everyone calls him Mitch), was desperately searching the medical literature for information because after six long months of a mysterious debilitating illness, his 12-year-old son's ailment had finally been diagnosed as Lyme disease. Despite aggressive treatment with the most advanced, sophisticated antibiotics available, his son was not recovering. A previously healthy, athletic boy, he could only walk with assistance when not in his wheelchair.

In one of Mitch's medical journals, he found a description of the experimental study Dr. William P. Fife was doing at Texas A&M University on the anaerobic spirochete that causes Lyme disease, an illness causing severe influenza-like symptoms. Mitch immediately called Dr. Fife, asking that his son be included in the non-responding Lyme disease study.

Mitch's son and two other Chico boys who were ill and showing the same symptoms were accepted in Dr. Fife's study. Oxygen under pressure accomplished what the most sophisticated drugs available had failed to achieve. After thirty treatments, the three boys were once again feeling well, walking, biking, and running like normal fourteen-year-old boys.

Mitch was so impressed by the success of this new and novel oxygen therapy that under the direction of and with the assistance of Dr. Fife, who had been a hyperbaric medicine pioneer in the United States, he and a group of his friends banded together to establish a hyperbaric clinic in Chico. They believed that HBO should be available to everyone in this northern California community.

On the day I telephoned to ask for details about chronic stroke recovery, Mitch told me his son was out playing football.

When we arrived at the Hyperbaric Center, John and I entered a reception office with the usual desk, couch, couple of chairs, and coffee table. Looseleaf notebooks filled with articles about Lyme disease and cerebral palsy were piled beside a few magazines.

Chris, one of the hyperbaric therapists, hurried out to meet us. She checked to be sure I was wearing all-cotton clothing before she led us down a hallway with offices on either side, into the Great Room. It was clear that life at the Chico Hyperbaric Clinic was centered around the large room at the far end of the hall.

The first thing I saw, filling one entire corner of the room, was an enormous white metal box that looked almost like one of those huge refrigerated trucks you pass on the freeway. This was the hyperbaric chamber itself, with a cheerful undersea mural of Disney-like fish on the side facing the room. There was a ramp leading up to the entrance of the six-person chamber, and a large round door that looked like the watertight door on a ship that opened onto the large tank. Inside the "tank" were facilities for six people, plus space for the hyperbaric attendant.

In the rest of the Great Room, there were low tables, each with four chairs. I saw jugs of bottled water beside a water cooler, a sink, and a refrigerator. It was a friendly space for friends and caregivers to wait while those being treated were in "the tank."

On that first day, there were four in the chamber, but only three of us being treated; Chuck, a stroke victim; four-and-a-half-year-old Timmie, being treated for cerebral palsy, accompanied by his father; and me.

Days later I was given a tour of the heart of "the works." The entire facility was not very complicated. Chris showed me an enormous tank, maybe eight feet tall, containing the pure oxygen in a storage room behind the Great Room. The oxygen tank was huge, cold—thick with frost—and it almost touched the ceiling. I saw pipes and assorted tubes and wires leading to and from the chamber, along with the tools needed for running this establishment. It wasn't nearly as complex as an MRI machine, which our local hospital *does* have.

Before my first "dive," Chris explained the safety regulations, as she did to each new patient: oxygen is a potentially flammable substance, so only cotton clothing is allowed in the chamber. Nothing greasy is permitted—no make-up, no perfume, hair spray, deodorant, wigs, or jewelry. Watches and fountain pens must be removed (the pressure could damage a watch or cause a pen to leak).

After she'd checked my blood pressure, a precaution she followed before every "dive," and I'd been fitted with a wide blue latex collar, we hyperbaric patients took our shoes off and walked in our cotton socks up the ramp to the loading platform. (Chuck was pushed in his wheelchair.)

Once on the platform, I was reminded of the heavy steel doors on a ship we'd visited when the Navy was in town, and the public had been invited aboard. Chris unlatched the massive round door (which I now saw had a VERY high threshold) and we climbed (Chuck was lifted) into the huge steel tank. Each side of the institutional-green chamber held three chairs with boldly checked black and white cushions. Looking at the domed ceiling, I was struck by the chamber's sturdy construction.

Chris was wearing casual navy cotton sweats. Although I was the only newcomer, she carefully explained the terminology and the procedure. Each session is called a "dive," a left-over term from hyperbaric oxygen's early days, when oxygen's only use was treating "the bends." We were going to be

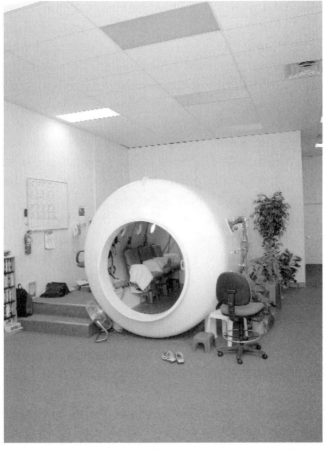

Hyperbaric chamber known as a multiplace chamber as it can accomodate more than one patient.

pressurized, or "going down," to the equivalent of twenty feet below sea level.

Chris warned us to let her know *IMMEDIATELY* if we felt pain in our ears while the pressure in the tank was being increased, and she told us to say "stop" if we did. "Don't try to be a tough guy. We can control the pressure, to give your ears time to adjust. We don't want any ruptured eardrums."

173

Blankets were stacked on one of the chairs inside the tank, but it was a warm November day and nobody asked for one. There were bright blue flexible plastic oxygen intake and vent tubes in the wall above each chair. One of the empty chairs held the clear, plastic hoods that were clamped onto our blue latex collars as soon as we were "down." Chris showed us the interior camera, mounted on one end of the chamber, that allowed the outside technician who controlled the pressure to keep an eye on us, just in case a medical problem should develop.

I didn't think to ask what medical emergencies they expected. Later I learned that children with very severe cerebral palsy have sometimes been known to respond to the increased pressure by regurgitating. Epileptic seizures have, rarely, been triggered by increased oxygen. None of these happened during any of my dives, but the attendants were prepared.

The door was latched, and I could hear air rushing into the tank. We were about fifteen feet "down" when I had to reluctantly admit I was feeling an ache in one ear. "It isn't bad," I protested, but Chris immediately called "stop" to the outside technician.

"Hold your nose and blow," she suggested, and showed me the technique, but I must be a slow learner. I held first one nostril and then the other. I blew and blew but nothing happened. I couldn't relieve the pressure. "Try swallowing," she suggested, and I tried to force a dry swallow. No luck. "How about some water," she asked, and handed me a bottle of chilled water. "Try drinking." So I chug-a-lugged and the pain in my ear vanished. "All clear now," she called to the outside technician. "We're ready to go on down," and once again I heard the sound of air flowing. I never did learn to "blow" to clear my ears, so for the next month I increased my water consumption by two chilled bottles a day.

It took about ten minutes to reach the desired atmospheric pressure, or "depth," or equivalent to approximately twenty feet below sea level. As soon as we were "down," Chris slipped one of the waiting transparent plastic hoods, about two feet tall and two feet wide, onto the individually fitted, blue latex collar each patient was wearing before she turned the oxygen on.

This was *it*. I knew pure oxygen was flowing into the hood, but there was no smell. No taste. It felt as if I was just breathing normal air. Chris, a registered nurse, sat beside the door, alert to each person's needs and meticulously checking the oxygen gages and our hoods during the hour, to be sure the correct pressure was maintained. Talking sounded a bit muffled inside the hood, although the conversation flowed easily. Each session lasted an hour, and she told us we were free to read, although the light was too dim to make reading comfortable. She suggested that we could doze, talk, or watch a video to wile away the hour. The Chico group has a video library, and tapes can be projected onto a small screen at the far end of the tank.

This was my first experience with a cerebral palsy child. For Timmie, the little four-year-old boy, it was wiggle, wiggle, wiggle. His father patiently held the child on his lap while Timmie did his darnedest to squirm away. He tried repeatedly to pull the oxygen hose off his hood. Briefly, he looked at family photos that his father had brought to amuse the boy, and he eventually settled down in Chris's lap while she told him about her son who was just about Timmie's age. It was a good thing that the hoses channeling oxygen into the hoods were both long and flexible. Chris hugged him, told him stories, and sang to him, quieting him for a moment, then he squirmed and wiggled even harder.

Timmie's father told me this was the first day of a new series of twenty treatments for his son. He'd had forty treatments during the past summer, and had improved so dramatically that he was back for forty more. His dad said the boy's vocabulary had greatly increased, as had his walking and muscular coordination.

During our hour, Timmie was one *extremely* active little boy. He managed to pull the tubes out of his plastic hood at least four times, and he loved the magnified echo of his hoots, shouts, and screams, enhanced and reverberating as they did inside the steel tank. He whipped through his father's supply of family snapshots at least five times, alternately kissing and kicking the photographed faces through his plastic hood, and good-naturedly tussling with his father and with Chris. Good thing his oxygen hose was at least eight feet long.

I'd been warned I might feel a tingling in my fingers and toes from the increased oxygen in my blood. No tingles. But when we came back "up" to normal air pressure, my ears crackled and popped like crazy, although I felt no pain. As soon as we were back in the Great Room, Chris carefully examined them. No redness. No problem.

176

"You might feel hungry," she'd warned me. "The oxygen stimulates your metabolism. If you get hungry, go ahead and eat." Half an hour later I realized she was so right. I was starving. After an "early" lunch (10:30 in the morning), I felt energized enough to investigate the borrowed laptop I'd brought, but had been too lethargic to open during the past week. An hour later, I was sleepy, so I took a nap. Back at 2:00 P.M. for my second round.

The hyperbaric staff: Chris is a caring, thirty-ish, brown-eyed blonde who'd earned her nursing degree from Butte Community College. During that first week she was seemingly tireless, holding Timmie on her lap, playing with him and singing songs to him. I met Karen, a pretty blond nurse-technician who'd trained under Dr. Fife, the man who pioneered the Lyme disease research at Texas A & M. And there was Mary, a tall brunette who usually ran the outside controls. I've also seen two young men, paramedic ambulance attendants who occasionally worked as "dive" technicians.

That first afternoon:

I was walking with less of a limp. My omnipresent, unsteady lack of balance was less noticeable, and the muscles in my right (affected) leg seemed more flexible. Overall, I felt better—more normal. This surprised me. I hadn't expected to see any results for at least two weeks. Maybe I was experiencing that "four hour buzz" I'd read about in one of the hyperbaric oxygen papers, and it was mighty welcome. What's next?

The afternoon stint was pretty much like the morning session. Timmie energetically wrestled with his dad for the entire hour. He was determined to remove his hood or yank out the oxygen intake tube or just yell and yell and yell. Maybe he was energized, too, by this morning's session.

What will he be like tomorrow? I'd never seen a child with cerebral palsy before, and I didn't know what to expect. I later learned that, like stroke victims, every child is different. Many are "too quiet," and Timmy's energy was welcomed by his incredibly patient father.

What will another pressurized oxygen session do for me?

That afternoon I felt a bit dazed when we "came back up" to standard air. Tired. No more new, good changes. Well, the morning improvements had surprised me and pleased me. I knew I shouldn't expect any changes during this first week while my brain begins to build new connections. Early to bed. Slept very well.

Tuesday, November 2:

Woke up early this morning. What did I expect after falling asleep about 9:30 last night? Wiggled my weak right arm and fingers. I do believe I can sense a subtle limbering of my hand. Walking seems easier, my right foot not catching on the carpet, so I guess it's not dragging.

No changes after this afternoon's "dive."

Wednesday, November 3:

Really tired after this morning's session. The muscles around my mouth are stiff and sluggish again, the way they were on a bad day after my stroke. Came home and slept for an hour, then woke up starving. What's going on inside my head? Last night my ear was quite painful. Better after a couple of acetamenophens. I'm managing to climb my daughter Sue's stairs more easily. The right knee still clicks with every "down" step, but it doesn't hurt. I guess that means it's no longer inflamed. Walking upstairs was difficult because I was tired, but each step felt easier. That unsteady, wiggling sensation in my head has returned.

Can it be that the nerves in my head are confused? I hope they're trying to rewire themselves into the old, normal patterns. If that's what's going on, this temporary stress will be well worth it. But yesterday and the day before my brain felt really clear, and it was so great to feel more "normal." We're off now for our morning walk in the park.

That afternoon:

After today's 2:00 P.M. session I asked one of the Lyme patients who was waiting for her next "dive" if it was normal to feel unusually tired. "Yes," she agreed, "Sometimes I do, too. It really 'takes it' out of you." No comment about "why" just breathing supplemental oxygen should exhaust me.

Not as tired this afternoon. Came home and rested, then wanted another walk in the park. My right leg is definitely behaving better. The muscles are more flexible and my stride, while still jerky, feels more natural. Going up and down the stairs to our bedroom is getting easier. I still have to use the banister to pull myself up, but now it's a one-handed effort, not the two-handed heave I used to haul myself up last Sunday when we arrived. No pain going downstairs, although the knee still clicks with every step. Head clear this afternoon. Wonderful to be free of that disturbing, unsteady tipping-back-and-forth lack of balance.

Thursday, November 4:

Seems as if every day is the same but different. Woke up with the same old buzz in my head, but I'm not exhausted the way I was yesterday morning. I do believe I have a bit more control of my right hand. I can almost wiggle my right fingers to match my left (good) hand. That numb, oblong patch on my lower forearm is less severe. When I left the hyperbaric facility this morning, all I wanted to do was walk in the park. I felt as if my body was saying, "Exercise, give me exercise," so that's what I'm going to do as soon as I finish this morning's notes.

My pals in the chamber:

Chuck is a stroke survivor too, but his stroke was a "bleed," far worse than mine. He's in a wheelchair and super unsteady, but he is able, with his wife's capable support and guidance, to shuffle the eight inches from the chamber hatch to his chair. Apparently he likes to read. He turns the pages of the motorcycle magazine he always brings, and when your hand is crippled it isn't easy to grasp and turn magazine pages. He understands what is said to him, but he can't speak, can't find the simplest words. I think the medical term for it is "aphasia."

Timmie was calmer today. He seems to be settling into the daily routine, which means alternating between wiggling and watching the video movie, depending on the show. He ignores cartoons and "talking heads," but loves adult splat-bash fights and car chases. He's starting to interact with Chuck and me, giving each of us a big grin and saying "Hi" over and over.

180

Friday, November 5:

A RED-LETTER DAY for Chuck.

He *walked* about three or four feet. He used a cane, and his steps were slow, shaky shuffles, but he *did* it. Big cheers all around from the staff and the rest of us— his wife, Timmie's father, and me. Chuck wore the biggest grin all afternoon and kept saying "Well! Well! Well!" Today he tried to answer one of Karen's questions, but couldn't find any word but "Well"; he's still having problems with word retrieval. He can repeat simple sentences when prompted by his wife Marilyn, but "Well" with varying intonations is his multipurpose answer to any question.

I woke up bright and early this morning, feeling terrific. Felt good all day. Energetic. Head almost clear. After the morning session, John and I went for our daily walk in the park. I left my husband sitting on a convenient bench beside the ½ mile marker because he was tired, but I walked almost twice as far as I had yesterday. I'll admit I was dragging (tired, *not* dragging my right foot) before we were home again, but I was ecstatic over having walked so much farther. I feel new strength and mobility in my right hand. Typing is faster and a tad more accurate. I haven't tried using my hand to write my name, but I'm afraid that skill hasn't returned yet. Will it ever?

Spent an hour at the clinic this morning after my "dive," reading their enormous file on Cerebral Palsy. So many enthusiastic comments from parents. And the thick binder on Lyme disease. HBO apparently works because the bacteria spewing out poisons in a Lyme disease victim's blood are anaerobic; oxygen kills the bacteria. Nothing on the coffee table about strokes. Karen says almost nothing has been written about strokes, which seems odd because they're so common, with many more victims than cerebral palsy, Lyme disease, or multiple sclerosis.

I can't help thinking about four million handicapped stroke survivors and their diminished lives in this year 1999.

11

THREE MORE WEEKS OF HBO

I've finished my first week at the clinic, and everyone takes Saturday and Sunday off. My son George and his daughters invited us to come down to Davis, a two hour drive south of Chico, for the weekend. It was a fine opportunity for a visit, and it will give Sue and her family a break from the old folks.

I'm curious. How much of my new energy is transient, a temporary gift of the daily high oxygen content I'm getting? How much will be permanent?

Week two.

Monday, November 8:

What a downer. I have my answer.

The weekend was strenuous, what with the drive down and back in California traffic, walking across three enormous grassy soccer fields the next morning to watch one granddaughter and her team play, and two full days with my hyperactive son, George, and his athletic girls. Just two days without extra oxygen running around in my veins had to be the equivalent of at least four normal days, and it's not permanent. At least, not yet.

This morning I felt the way I did before I started the treatments—all shaky and lacking in energy. My muscles were rigid and my speech dragged. I could talk, but slowly. I knew what I wanted to say, but I had to concentrate to make my tongue work. I felt slightly better after this morning's session.

We went to the park for our usual morning walk, but the muscles in my right leg were spastic. They refused to relax, and I was back to my old limping, stiff-muscled gait. Had to cry "uncle" when we reached the first bench. I was too tired to go farther. Not at all like last Friday when I walked all the way up to the bridge (about a mile) and back without being exhausted.

Our therapy group has grown and changed. Timmie has been shifted to another time slot (thank goodness) with several other brain-damaged children. I know I sound unsympathetic, but I was ignorant. He was the first cerebral palsied child I'd ever seen. I didn't realize that there are some parents of CP children who would be thrilled if their child was able to wiggle and scream.

I had a talk with Chuck's wife, Marilyn, this afternoon. He is only fifty-one. They have no idea what caused his stroke. He wasn't overweight. Didn't have high blood pressure or any of the usual pre-stroke health problems. His was a massive stroke, hemorrhagic, the kind that doctors routinely just "write off." He was completely helpless. Couldn't swallow. Couldn't move. She told me he had a series of sixty treatments last spring, and he had made such dramatic gains that they've come back for forty more.

They used to be professional musicians—she says he blew a mean trumpet, and she played the piano and sang. She brought an audio tape the other day so we could hear one of their performances, and I agree, Chuck did blow a clean, pure trumpet, and Marilyn had, and probably still has, a sexy, smoky voice. They live in a small town in the Sierras, about two hours from the clinic. She first heard about hyperbaric oxygen and this treatment center at a Christmas party.

We've been joined by two new stroke survivors. There was 80-year-old Frank, with a mischievous grin and a wink. He has bright blue eyes, lives here in town, speaks easily, but moves with extreme difficulty. V-e-r-y s-l-o-w-l-y. He and I agreed that, "life after a stroke isn't living, it's only 'existing.'"

Frank was on a gurney (bed), and the technicians had already removed two chairs from one side of the chamber so they could slide his gurney into the space against one wall. Mighty flexible.

I asked Frank's daughter, Erin, the usual question, "How did you find out about hyperbaric oxygen?" She'd searched the Internet, read about strokes being treated with HBO, and insisted that her Daddy try the treatment. Erin said he'd had his stroke several months ago, had forty treatments that helped him so much that she insisted he come back for a second round. She thinks many of his improvements are permanent, which made me feel better. She gave me copies of several papers she'd found on the Internet describing the improvements HBO had made in other chronic stroke victims. Today Frank dozed for the entire hour, and I soon learned that a nap was his every-day routine in the chamber.

Rosalie joined our group. She's a henna-haired seventy-four, and defiantly said she'd only agreed to "try" the oxygen treatments at the insistence of a relative, but she's sure nothing is going to change. "Not after four years," she announced firmly. Says she's only here to keep peace in the family. With that mind set, it will be interesting to see what the next three weeks will do for her.

Her stroke left her with a paralyzed left hand and two rigidly crossed fingers. She says she does all her own housework, and that the paralyzed hand doesn't keep her from playing cards with her friends. She's a widow, lives alone, walks easily, and drives herself to and from her home, which is seventeen miles from town. She has a penetrating voice, and she's a non-stop talker. She wasn't with us this afternoon. She has cautiously started with just one oxygen treatment a day.

I felt terrific after the afternoon's session. Big change from last night after we drove back from Davis, and I was so tired I could scarcely stay awake through dinner. Later, played Scrabble with my granddaughter, Summer, and daughter, Sue, then read until 9:30.

This may sound like "just another useless anecdote" to be scoffed at by physicians, but "quality of life" is important and mine has certainly improved. Life is great when you feel good.

Tuesday, November 9:

Chuck missed this morning's session—Marilyn has the 'flu.' There's a rule that's at least equal to Murphy's Law. Caregivers are 'not allowed' to be sick. She'd recovered enough this afternoon to drive him to the clinic and push his wheelchair up the ramp. My hat's off to caregivers. Theirs is a daunting, never-ending task. They deserve support and help from their friends and tons of respect. A stroke changes life for everyone in the family.

Frank slept peacefully in the "tank," and I drove home very thankful for my blessings, even if one of

George's daughters did say in my hearing, "Grandma talks as if her mouth is full of mush."

Friday, November 12:

Today I almost felt as if I'd recovered from my stroke. It was glorious. Still two more weeks of treatments. Oh, I hope these good changes are permanent. That they won't depend on getting constant boosters of oxygen.

Monday, November 15th, starting my third week:

We spent this weekend quietly with the family. Rosalie has joined Chuck, Frank, and me to make a twice-a-day foursome in the chamber.

Can't help wondering what changes I'll see this week. Will Rosalie still complain about her sore bum because she has to sit for an entire hour? Will Chuck still be "reading" his motorcycle magazines? Marilyn says he is not really reading, just looking at the pictures, but she thinks/hopes he is on the verge of being able to read again. And to talk. I hope so, too. His vocabulary still consists of "well," with various intonations.

Tuesday, November 16:

Each day seems to be the same as the day before, yet different. Hard for me to see further new changes. I've decided it's like watching a baby grow. When you see the child all day, every day, you don't notice the little changes, just the 'big' things, like creeping, then crawling, and finally taking those first tottering steps. People who haven't seen the infant for a month or so, however, always comment on, "How much he's grown" or "Goodness, how she's changed."

I've worked up to a mile and a half on our daily walks in the park, and John has also increased his distance a bit. He now walks as far as the second picnic bench where he sits, enjoying the sunshine and the fall colors while he waits for me. I try to go a little farther each day. Some days I seem to be easily striding along, other days the right leg muscles stiffen up, bringing back the old lurch-and-stride.

I had an interesting experience one night this week. One of Sue's friends, a physical therapist, stopped by for a visit. Sue's a nurse, and her friends have been curious about the new "experimental" treatment her mom has been taking. The physical therapist asked how I was doing and challenged me to try the "standing on one leg" test again. I'd tried it a week ago and could only stand alone on my weak right leg for a single second. Last night I stood stork-legged on my right foot for four seconds, and I could actually feel the calf muscles in my leg responding while I swayed. First time I've felt those muscles move since the stroke. Of course, the first time the PT tested me, I'd had half a beer, and last night I was sipping a soft drink. Maybe that had something to do with the improvement, but I did feel a new response in those reluctant muscles.

Last night Sue and I were fixing dinner together, and she told me she'd been talking with one of the physicians at her hospital—a doctor who occasionally sends a patient for hyperbaric treatment, usually for Lyme disease. "Why don't you send your stroke patients," she'd asked. The doctor answered, "Oh, sometimes that treatment works for strokes. Sometimes it doesn't."

Sometimes it works, and sometimes it doesn't!

I stared at her, appalled. "What is that doctor saying? Doesn't he know there's no drug or treatment that always works for everyone? Not even good old, dependable, time-tested aspirin? That's why drug companies have to tell you every possible side effect of every product they market."

It was hard for me to believe that any doctor could know there was a chance hyperbaric oxygen would help someone who'd had a stroke, but wouldn't give his patient the option of making up his or her own mind about trying it. (At the patient's own expense, regardless of how much medical insurance they held.)

Sue doesn't give up easily. "But if it works for some stroke victims," she'd persisted, "why is it so hard for them to find out about hyperbaric oxygen therapy?"

"Oh, we expect people to hear about it by word of mouth. Of course, the insurance companies won't touch it, because the hyperbaric providers can't guarantee results." And he went on to tell her, "There are a few places down in southern California that offer it, but they're very expensive, with physicians on staff, physical therapy facilities, nutrition guidance, and the whole ball of wax."

When she repeated that man's casual statement about his patients having to live a handicapped life because their physician wouldn't tell them about an alternative, and they hadn't heard the latest gossip, I couldn't help snapping, "But it's his responsibility to give his patients the option of trying anything that may work. Why can't he just say, 'Sometimes it works miracles, sometimes it doesn't help at all'? Let his patient make the choice."

"Hey, Mom," she said quietly. "I'm just a nurse, and he's a doctor. We don't tell doctors how to treat their patients. It just isn't done."

I said, "Mitch's place is right here in town, and it isn't all that fancy. I know there are some elegant hyperbaric facilities in Southern California that are set up in expensive, spa-like surroundings where they treat the whole patient with pressurized oxygen, electrical stimulation, diet modification, and extensive physical therapy. After all, it is southern California. And wealthy stroke victims have a right to receive the finest and most complete restorative care available, don't they? If they have a stroke, they're just as disabled as the rest of us. They hurt just as much. Are just as awkward. Just as frustrated.

"But most of the hyperbaric places I found on the Internet charge just what we're paying here."

"I know, Mom," she said with a smile, her voice soothing. "Now don't get your blood pressure up. Just keep your diary. And if these treatments help you, tell everyone you know."

I couldn't stop arguing. This was so important. "But for the ordinary stroke victim like me," I stormed, "someone who just wants to get his or her life back and can't afford luxurious pampering, there are thirteen free-standing hyperbaric clinics in southern California. And most of them cost exactly what we're paying Mitch.

"If your doctor sends his Lyme patients to Mitch's clinic, he should know that HBO helps people recover from strokes. Mitch's, and these other clinics, do help people who only need (or can only afford) daily oxygen to help them recover from a stroke, or to control their multiple sclerosis, or to help children with cerebral palsy like Timmie, or someone with a brain injury. Not just," I added, "to treat Lyme disease."

I jabbed my finger at the list I'd been working on that afternoon. "There's nothing fancy or 'alternative' about oxygen. Doesn't he know the FDA, the AMA, and Medicare all approved pressurized oxygen for:

Air or gas embolism
Carbon monoxide poisoning and smoke inhalation
Carbon monoxide poisoning complicated by
    cyanide poisoning
Clostridial myonecrosis (gas gangrene)
Crush injury compartment syndrome and other
    acute traumatic ischemias
Decompression sickness (the Bends)
Enhancement of healing in selected problem
    wounds
Exceptional blood loss (anemia)
Necrotizing soft tissue infections
Osteomyelitis (refractory)
Radiation tissue damage (osteoradionecrosis)
Skin grafts and flaps (compromised)
Thermal burns."

"He knows, Mom." She walked over to me and put her arms around me. "I know how frustrating it must be for you. Here you are working so hard to recover from your stroke, and you're doing so much better. You just want the whole world to know about it. To use it."

"Of course I do," I agreed. It helped, knowing Sue understood why I was so upset, but I couldn't stop arguing, justifying my anger. "Edward Teller says it's 'good science,' and there are so many people who can be helped."

The next morning I was still steaming a bit. I think it is wicked. Immoral. Unethical for anyone in the medical profession to withhold information from four million handicapped Americans just because the treatment doesn't always work for everyone. To not tell patients about the possibility of improving the quality of their lives! To condemn victims of Lyme disease to pain-filled lives in wheelchairs if they don't happen to live here. To not tell multiple sclerosis victims that they could slow down the progress of their disease. Or to refuse to treat children with cerebral palsy with oxygen, just because their parents haven't heard the right gossip.

Wednesday, November 17:

I'm half way through my third week, and I'm depressed. I haven't felt any new, spectacular improvements. Monday I was very tired after both the morning and afternoon sessions. Restless. Slept badly. Felt disorganized. Not "confused," just "not quite with it" after the morning "dive."

I keep telling myself the nerve cells in my brain are trying to reestablish their old patterns. To do this, they have to reorganize themselves, change the unsatisfactory, makeshift patterns they've cobbled together. One of the things I've learned about human beings is that we do try to adapt to whatever situation we're in. My brain must be very busy making all those changes.

I know I'm climbing the stairs more easily—not hauling myself up, hand over hand on the banister the way I did the first week we were here. Last week I was using only one hand for balance and stepping more easily. My speech seems more fluid, but it's hard to measure tiny changes on a day-to-day basis.

Yesterday Marilyn told me about Chuck's daily physical therapy workout. After the morning "dive," he spends a couple of hours exercising—that means standing up, sitting down, taking steps, sitting in a chair, and getting up again. I know these exercises sound simplistic, but for a stroke-damaged person, that's an exhausting routine.

He's determined he will recover, and I've seen big improvements in the last two weeks. This morning, after Marilyn had gently coached him, he was able to repeat in soft tones, "G o o d... m o r n i n g... P o l l y." I was so thrilled I wanted to kiss him.

Rosalie's hands don't look as if they're hurting, and her left hand seems to be more relaxed, except for those two rigidly crossed fingers. She didn't say how she was feeling, and I didn't ask. After she'd been so adamant about "no change is possible," how could she admit she was feeling better?

Thursday the 19th:

No depression today. I woke up feeling new strength. Not exactly surges of energy, just a basic return to normal.

Week four, Wednesday, November 24:

For some reason, I've been exhausted all week. Fatigued on Monday. Tired Tuesday, but felt better after the afternoon session. Talking seems to come and go—jaw and tongue still tight at night when I'm tired, but almost normal when I'm fresh.

Thursday, November 25:

Tomorrow is my last day.

Chuck has gone home. Finished his four weeks. For a man who was "written off" by his doctors, Marilyn says he has literally "come back to life." Last Friday he walked all the way from the front door, down the hall, and into the "Great Room." He's far more alert than he was two weeks ago, and his eyes are bright and happy. He wants to talk, knows what he wants to say, but so far, "well, well, well" is all that comes out, with different tones for different meanings. He is processing information—it's just that he still can't find the words. Marilyn is convinced that he's on the brink of speech recovery.

Rosalie has certainly perked up. Her left hand is slowly uncurling, although she says she still can't use it. I think she's forgotten that she has a left hand. Her mental attitude has improved. She continues to insist that after having had a stroke four years ago, she's going to have all of her problems for the rest of her life, but she's far more relaxed and alert. No speech problems for her. She walks easily, talks easily and constantly.

Frank is beginning to move his "useless" leg, although he can't lift it easily, and his left hand is still utterly useless. He's very alert mentally and has a great smile. Erin says he was seriously depressed after his stroke, which was only four months ago. I can certainly understand that.

I am walking far more easily, although my right leg muscles still stiffen up when I'm tired. Talking is easier, and I'm told the "droop" on the right side of my face has almost disappeared. Hooray for that. I have tons more energy, although I still fall asleep at 9:30 every night. No need for naps though.

During these last two weeks I've felt a bit disoriented after an hour in the chamber, although my head clears up later. I wonder if that is one of the effects of oxygen. Now I'll be watching and waiting for those promised six months or more of improvement while my brain continues to grow sturdy new blood capillaries to feed all my newly awakened neurons.

12

HEALING IS HARDER THAN IT SOUNDS

The third of February, 2000. It's been 9 weeks since we returned from Chico, and I have to admit the first seven or eight have been tough. Within a week of getting home I was losing many of the benefits I'd felt in Chico.

Sure, many of my dormant cells had been active while they were getting their daily oxygen "fix," but there hadn't been time for my body to build a set of sturdy new blood vessels. Now they were going back to sleep. I hadn't yet read Dr. Jain's chapter describing "stroke" and oxygen's role in rehabilitating the ischemic penumbra:

1. Unmasking or release from inhibition of previously non-functioning pathways
2. Synaptic sprouting and formation of new dendritic connections for pathways for transmission of neural messages

I didn't know whether I was feeling so sluggish and tired because I was fatigued after the five hour drive home, or because I was coming down with a cold. After we'd been home for four days, while I was taking my morning shower, I realized a muscle in my right buttock was getting hard and stiff again.

"Oh, no," I thought. Is the limp coming back? I fervently hoped it would go away, but it didn't. Every morning after that I checked my right buttock and could feel more of my muscles becoming rigid or spastic. I was limping again. And the old backward and forward unsteadiness was returning. Did this mean I'd lost all the benefits of HBO? That those wonderful improvements weren't permanent? Were they all going to melt away without a constant fresh supply of pressurized oxygen?

In September and October, I'd been so excited over the possibility of regaining some control of my body that I'd skipped right over that ugly word "regression" while reading those enthusiastic reports and arranging my Chico visit. I hadn't read those upbeat hyperbaric messages carefully enough, blithely skipping over such phrases as "rebuilding of capillaries" and ignoring the fact that it takes time, lots of time, to rebuild and rewire neuronal connections.

In the stabilized stroke the main function of pressurized oxygen is the rebuilding of capillaries, relieving the hypoxia, reducing brain edema or swelling, restoring the integrity of the damaged cell membranes, and neutralizing the toxic waste products.

I tried to tell myself my cold was rotten, getting Christmas presents bought, wrapped, and mailed to the kids was stressful, and the weather was cold and rainy. Those had to be the reason I was feeling so "down." But when friends who knew we'd been gone for a month and that I was going to try a wonderful

198

new kind of stroke rehabilitation, came up with cheerful faces and asked, "How did it go," I squirmed and temporized, saying "The jury is still out, but I know that I'm better."

Truthfully, I was beginning to wonder. Was it really worth all that time and money? I honestly didn't feel as good as I had in October.

There were improvements I could measure, but I wasn't walking as far or as easily as I'd done in Chico. I was limping again, although I *could* walk farther than I had been able to last August. My handwriting was just a smidgen better, still jagged and jiggly, but I could make it stay on a single line, and I was able to read the grocery notes I so laboriously drew. My signature began to look almost like an adult's, but real handwriting was still beyond me. Thank heavens for the computer keyboard. I could send e-mails to the kids, and type two- or three-line greetings on our Christmas cards to old friends.

I re-read every scrap of material that I'd printed from the Internet and tried to reinforce my "I really am getting better" attitude because the experts all agreed that improvements continue for six months or longer.

When I sent a plaintive query to the HBO chat-line asking about regression, I received several up-beat answers reassuring me with success stories (after 80 or 100 treatments) and suggesting that I return for more. At the time, this was not an option. I was just going to have to admit that at my age it was ridiculous to whine about being handicapped.

The HBO providers actually had written about regression in veiled terms, but I hadn't read carefully enough. Let me say in their defense, it's probably a matter of follow-up. These HBOT physicians have seen remarkable improvements in their patients while they were getting daily oxygen. It was only later, after we'd gone home, that the slump hit. It's devastating, having those newly regained abilities vanish again.

But every day I felt a bit weaker and I was so tired all the time. For the next six weeks my blood pressure jumped around like a yo-yo—sometimes as high as 195 and sometimes as low as 119. Without commenting on or asking about the HBO experience (my regular doctor was too tactful to say "I told you so"), he increased my medication, and the blood pressure finally steadied. Taking those strong, expensive pills instead of pressurized oxygen annoyed me, because I knew my blood pressure had been rock-solid normal during all of November. A standard part of the daily routine had been recording each patient's blood pressure before every "dive," and my systolic numbers had been so normal—125 to 136, some mornings as low as 110.

Those 195 figures frightened me. Led to my thinking I would probably have another stroke, and I certainly didn't want *that.* Never again. If I *did* have another stroke, and I knew that strokes are the third leading cause of death, I hoped the next one would end this exhausting, never-ending struggle. In fact, dying was a very attractive option. No wonder "depression" is so common in stroke patients. There were days when I felt so lethargic that I just babied myself and read all day, except for clumsily preparing our meals, and those had been remarkably simplified.

It was getting harder and harder to speak. The right side of my face seemed to freeze up. I couldn't make my tongue work properly, and when I did try to talk, I could feel my lip being pulled out of shape. My words sounded distorted, at least to me, although when I complained, friends would say, "No, no, you're speaking very well." But I could hear myself speaking, and I didn't like what I heard. For most of the month of November I'd been talking reasonably easily and clearly, although on a few evenings, after I'd had a very active day, the left side of my face had felt stiff.

I remember playing Trivia one night with twelve-year-old April and her girlfriend. They insisted that I read most of the questions aloud. I'd walked a long way that day, beyond the bridge, and I was tired. Reading those questions was a struggle, because my mouth wasn't working properly that night, but the girls were showing me "tough love." They knew speaking aloud was good therapy, and they wouldn't let me quit. Now it was happening all the time.

A recent television ad for car insurance showed a junkyard filled with crumpled cars. The announcer had it right. "The cars are the lucky ones. They can be thrown away. It's the damaged people who have to struggle on."

I found the answer one morning on the chat-line. A woman had written to Dr. James, asking:

Why do you think Ben does great during treatments and then goes into this backward slide as soon as they are stopped? For about a month, he becomes confused again (more than before his treatments) and then starts to improve again. Is it

201

another clearing stage he is going through? He definitely is improving because of his HBOT treatments. Is there something else we could do for him until he starts HBOT again?

So it wasn't just me. It happened to other stroke survivors, too. She was asking the questions I wanted answered, but she'd had the good sense to write directly to Dr. James, the Scottish hyperbaric expert, instead of questioning an entire chat-line. His reply explained why I was feeling so rotten.

Recovery is complex, but there are two factors that are probably involved in this effect. The blood vessels in the nervous system are different from those in the rest of the body because of the need to protect the very sensitive nerve tissue from many components of blood that are toxic.

The lining cells of the blood vessels—from the large arteries (the carotids), down to the smallest draining veins (capillaries)—form a barrier known as the blood-brain barrier. This has not interested neurologists very much but has been studied in detail by the drug industry because of the need to get drugs past the barrier. We know little about repair mechanisms for the blood-brain barrier, but we know that it does repair itself.

I stared at Dr. James' answer. So that's what the medics mean when they talk about the "blood-brain barrier." I had wondered what the barrier was. Now I knew. It's a special lining in the brain's delivery system. That's a very clever bit of engineering by the Creator.

202

I was happy to see that Dr. James says the lining does repair itself. His answer continues:

> *Oxygen therapy allows new capillaries to form in the damaged tissue, but this is a slow process. It starts because of the extra oxygen made available under hyperbaric conditions. The daily HBOT was probably keeping the swelling in check, but when it is stopped, the swelling increases until the new capillary growth is eventually able to restore a more normal tissue content.*
>
> *Best wishes,*
> *Philip James*

I heaved a great sigh of relief. Yes, that had to be the answer. The swelling in my brain really had temporarily returned when it was no longer getting the oxygen it needed, but that is a normal part of the process. Dr. James didn't say "how long" it takes for the blood brain barrier to repair itself; he'd simply said the body does make those necessary repairs. As soon as the new capillaries are securely in place, the improvements will be permanent.

And I came across another juicy little tidbit.

> *The human brain contains something like ten billion neurons and about a hundred billion synapses. We know these neurons communicate chemically and electrically with each other in multiple ways via these contact points...*
>
> Jackson, Gabe; *Civilization and Barbarity*
> Humanity Books, 1999.

Rebuilding even a minute portion of ten billion neurons: that is a "WOW" figure to play with.

And I was disappointed because I'd expected several million neurons to function as well as they had while I was temporarily giving my brain all the pressurized oxygen it needed. I know I have a bunch of sleeping neurons, and I know they're perfectly willing to become active again because they did perk up while they were receiving supplemental oxygen. But there hasn't been enough time for a new set of capillaries and their specialized "delivery" tubes to rebuild themselves.

But I couldn't help thinking, and I'll admit it makes me very angry, that if the medical world wasn't so focused on man-made "cures" *after* the damage is done, I wouldn't have to go through these difficult spells. Just giving me ordinary unpressurized oxygen to prevent the secondary swelling while I was having this "minor" stroke may have prevented almost all of the damage I've been working so hard to overcome.

While I was searching for information about "regression," I came across one of those "help yourself to health" articles answering a question a reader had asked about the new "oxygen therapy." The good doctor said he was "unaware of any medical centers using this technique" and finished his article saying "the problem is that the growth of brain cells is slow, only a millimeter or two a week, so progress occurs glacially." This was hardly a "keep on trying" bit of advice I needed or wanted.

The suggestions from another stroke victim were just what I needed to hear:

Go for a daily walk if you are no longer receiving therapy. Count the blocks or the telephone poles to measure how far you've walked, and to exercise the "remembering" part of your brain. Do not get lazy. Use a cane if you need it but forget the wheelchair. Your atrophy needs the blood flow.

Maintain your hygiene. You just might bump into a friend or special person who sees you and is inspired by your efforts.

Think positively. Keep trying to move a paralyzed limb even when you "know" it won't budge. If you don't involve it, your paralyzed part will think you don't need it anymore. This is the basis of the new "restraint" therapy.

Be sure to take your meds every day for stroke prevention—aspirin, Coumadin, or Warfarin— whatever your doctor suggests.

Use gardening or whatever hobby tickles your fancy. You can grow roses or pansies, or try a new recipe with just one side of your body.

Exercise your brain every day—if you have access to a computer, use it to search for facts, to stay in touch with your friends or family and write down the URLs (sites) as you go. Quiz yourself at the end of each day. This tells your brain that "remembering" is important. That you need more space on the brain's "hard drive."

I hadn't realized it when I started writing this book, but searching the web and typing each chapter has actually been "good therapy" for me, stimulated and reinforced by my determination to share everything I've learned about strokes.

January 23. My birthday.

A funny thing has been happening. Slowly, some of the improvements I'd felt in Chico have begun to return. Time was the key. Time and exercise.

We live on a steep hill. The street is icy in December, so the city spreads cinders to provide traction for cars. Walking on cinder-strewn asphalt isn't very smart. It's tricky and dangerous, almost like walking on ball-bearings, so I'd been getting very little exercise during the month of December. Just an occasional short stroll when we drove down to the park, maybe once a week, or sometimes limping the necessary two or three blocks when I had to do some shopping.

We joined the 'Y' early in January and began swimming every day, and that's made all the difference. I started out safely enough, using only the breast stroke so I could keep my head above water, cautiously swimming beside the wall in case I got into trouble. But today I was able to flutter-kick for the first time. I could feel the muscles in my right leg almost doing what I asked them to do. I'd tried several times earlier this month, and my right leg had feebly wiggled maybe five or six times before it quit, while my left leg fluttered away at the well-remembered eight times a stroke. Darned lopsided, and each time I tried the standard crawl, I ended up sputtering with my face full of water.

But today things changed. My right leg was moving, weakly I'll admit, but it *moved* the entire length of the pool. My brain really was doing what HBO had promised. It was growing new connections. I asked my right leg to kick, and it kicked! Proof that things were starting to get back to normal.

Three Years Later

Home from Chico after a second set of forty HBO treatments. I'm feeling alive, and it's wonderful. No more jiggly, backward-and-forward struggle for balance every time I stand or take a step. No more rigid facial muscles when I'm tired and can't make my face work and my tongue won't form the words. I can even have a conversation again with my husband and with friends, or on the telephone. True, I'm still limping, but the muscles in my right leg don't get stiff until late in the day. My handwriting is still slow and laborious, but I *can* take a message or fill out a simple form. I no longer have to humiliate myself by saying, "Sorry. I can't write."

I've learned a lot about strokes. I'm living proof that more *can* be done, that more *should* be done and that hyperbaric oxygen is effective. The sooner it is given the better, but HBO can do a great deal to heal the nerve damage, even years later.

The Year 2004

The above was written before I began regressing again. Physicians seldom see what happens to patients after they are no longer getting a daily oxygen "fix."

The brain swelling returns, almost as if a "new" injury had occurred, but angiogenesis has been going on for a month, which means many new capillaries are in place. These fresh young blood vessels are sturdy and allow oxygen-carrying red blood cells to feed many more brain cells, but they don't reach all of them.

It's been almost exactly six years since I was felled by that damnable, cussed stroke, and it's been a roller-coaster of an existence. What have I learned?

I've never forgotten the moment when one of the hospital nurses said in a soothing voice as she helped me into the bathroom, "Just think of this as taking a different path in your life's journey."

A different path!

It's been that. The landscape of my life has changed from that of a normal, placid world holding only the usual aging problems into a parched hillside filled with rocks for me to stumble over or bark my shins on. It's a new world filled with crags I can't climb, gullies I can't leap over, and underfoot there is only an occasional clump of bleached dry grass.

Fatigue is a constant. This seems to be a frequent complaint among stroke survivors, one common to all the people I've met on the stroke chat-line. I'm always tired. Have to push myself to do even the simplest necessary tasks. I try to understand this constant fatigue and imagine that the demands I now place on the undamaged nervous tissues that I have left creates such a burden that those nerves are exhausted. They simply can not move the muscles they once commanded. And of course, unused muscles atrophy. All I know for sure is that my thigh muscles ache constantly—a situation that has led to less and less exercise, and less exercise has led to muscles that complain, even when I'm sitting still.

Walking is no longer a matter of swinging along with pleasure. It's a troublesome effort that requires thought and determination with every step. Talking is equally problematic. I can usually *answer* the telephone and speak clearly, but if I am asked to initiate a phone call, just that tiny amount of stress makes my facial muscles stiffen up.

Were the results of the HBO treatments permanent? Some have been and that's great, but many of my disabilities have returned. They seem to come and go. Several HBO providers suggest that post-stroke patients have an HBO treatment every week or so to keep the improvements going.

Would I continue breathing oxygen under pressure if it were available? You bet I would. If I were Dr. Teller, the physicist, and I could afford to buy and maintain my own hyperbaric chamber, I would do as he does and spend one hour in it every other day. I would be constantly building new capillaries, growing more new brain cells. But I don't have the $60,000 or so that it would take to buy a used one, and I would still need a trained attendant to run it.

Or I would schedule a weekly treatment if a hyperbaric facility was available in our part of the state. No matter what the financial sacrifice, I would do whatever it took to avoid the bitter disappointments of regression—the returned clumsiness, the renewed aches and spasticity.

What I WOULD ask for, if I could ask the genie of the lamp for just a single wish, would be the recovery of all the brain cells that were not injured by that original miniscule clot. Had I been given oxygen during the first hours of the event, I probably would have no problems. By now I would have learned to accept and live with the minimal damage I sustained during those first hours. I've been cheered to learn that brains *do* know how to slowly heal themselves when the damage is not overwhelming.

I think the thing I miss more than anything else is the joy I used to feel in being alive—my family, my friends, my world. This began to fade about six months after the stroke when I slowly and reluctantly began to understand that I wasn't ever going to recover, no matter how diligently I tried. Exercise may be a part of the solution, but it is not the whole answer.

Yes, I do continue seeing miniscule permanent improvements, but I'm still messy at the table, dropping food on the floor despite trying to be careful. Yes, I can drive safely. The Oregon Department of Transportation has checked my physical and mental status and okayed me. Yes I can type—but my right hand insists upon "dancing" above the keyboard, and my two right middle fingers must still be individually "commanded" to tap the correct keys. Yes, I can speak most of the time, but I can't depend on either my lips or my tongue, and there are other, more intimate body functions that I cannot always control.

How can we convince the American medical industry to recognize use of this natural, elemental medical substance and to administer oxygen to oxygen-deprived tissues? If I had a simple answer to that question, I would already have acted.

It is unreasonable and unrealistic to expect every family in the U.S. to possess their own individual HBO chamber because oxygen has so many medical emergency uses, as well as healing chronic ailments. Nobody needs to or should use HBO all day, every day, because too much oxygen, like too much water or too much of anything, can do you no good. Nor do most of us have the training to use HBO equipment safely and responsibly. And we don't need to keep CAT scanning equipment handy in our homes. That equipment is, or should be, available in the hospital. It, too, requires a trained operator and should be used only when and where appropriate.

But it *is* reasonable to ask the medical community to focus on oxygen-replacement measures for hypoxic (oxygen-starved) tissues. The pharmaceutical world is unlocking medical mysteries at a breath-taking pace. At this time, researchers are investigating life on a molecule by molecule basis and learning the mechanics of disease-causing bacteria and viruses. Medical investigators are creating miracles of agricultural cloning, artificial insemination, and mechanical hearts. There are so many new horizons. There is plenty of space for innovative, profit-making biotechnology and authentic, profitable challenges toward the creation of a better, safer human environment.

We don't need to re-invent oxygen. Our problems start when the delivery system breaks down. I propose that the medical community stop tinkering with attempts to invent a new substitute for air. Let's recognize this natural, essential miracle and use it. Use our air the way we use water and soil for healthy, productive living.

211